Core Clinical Cases in Obstetrics and Gynaecology

Core Clincal Cases in Obstetrics and Gynaecology
A *problem-solving approach*

Janesh Kumar Gupta
MB ChB, MSc, MD, MRCOG

Clinical Senior Lecturer/Honorary Consultant in Obstetrics and Gynaecology, Module Co-ordinator for Undergraduate Obstetrics and Gynaecology Course at University of Birmingham Medical School, Academic Department of Obstetrics and Gynaecology, Birmingham Women's Hospital, Birmingham, UK

Gary Mires
MD, FRCOG

Senior Lecturer and Honorary Consultant, Department of Obstetrics and Gynaecology, Ninewells Hospital and Medical School, University of Dundee, Dundee, UK

Khalid Saeed Khan
MB BS, FCPS, MSc, MRCOG, Dip Med Ed

Consultant Obstetrician and Gynaecologist, Birmingham Women's Hospital, University of Birmingham, Birmingham, UK

A member of the Hodder Headline Group
LONDON
Distributed in the United States of America by
Oxford University Press Inc., New York

First published in Great Britain in 2001 by
Arnold, a member of the Hodder Headline Group,
338 Euston Road, London NW1 3BH

http://www.arnoldpublishers.com

Distributed in the USA by
Oxford University Press Inc.,
198 Madison Avenue, New York, NY10016
Oxford is a registered trademark of Oxford University Press

British Library Cataloguing in Publication Data
A catalogue record for this book is available from the British Library

Library of Congress Cataloging in Publication Data
A catalog record for this book is available from the Library of Congress

ISBN 0 340 76042 7

2 3 4 5 6 7 8 9 10

Typeset in 9.5pt on 12 pt Ocean Sans by Phoenix Photosetting, Chatham, Kent
Printed and bound in India by Replika Press Pvt. Ltd.

What do you think about this book? Or any other Arnold title?
Please send your comments to feedback.arnold@hodder.co.uk

Contents

Preface

Why *core* clinical cases?

In undergraduate medical education there is a trend towards the development of 'core' curricula. The aim is to facilitate the teaching of essential and relevant knowledge, skills and attitudes. This is in sharp contrast to traditional curricula, where there was an emphasis on detailed factual information, often without any practical clinical relevance. Currently, students' learning is being more commonly examined using objective structured clinical examinations which assess the practical use of knowledge, rather than the regurgitation of small-print information that was commonly emphasised in traditional examination methods. This book has defined the 'core' material for obstetrics and gynaecology by considering the common core clinical problems which may be encountered in primary and secondary care, and it provides a learning strategy to master this 'core' material for examinations.

Why a *problem-solving* approach?

In practice, patients present with clinical problems, which are explored through history, examination and investigation progressively leading from a differential to a definitive diagnosis. Unfortunately, standard textbooks tend to present the subject matter according to a pathophysiological classification which does not help to prepare students to confront clinical scenarios. We have therefore based this book on a problem-solving approach. This inculcates the capacity for critical thinking and helps students to analyse the basis of clinical problems. The deep understanding of learning issues acquired in this way means that knowledge can be more easily retrieved both to solve real patients' problems in the future and to answer confidently clinical questions encountered in examinations.

How will this book inspire problem-solving traits?

The short case scenarios presented in this book are based on common core clinical cases which students are likely to encounter in an undergraduate obstetrics and gynaecology module. We have grouped these cases according to areas of patients' complaints. There are seven groups in the gynaecology category and six groups in obstetrics. Each group includes five or six cases, which begin with a statement of the patient's complaint followed by a short description of the patient's problem. For each case, using a question and short answer format, the student is taken through a problem-solving exercise. There are two types of problem-solving cases in this book. One type deals with the development of a diagnostic and therapeutic strategy, and the other deals with the development of a counselling strategy. The sequence of the cases and questions in each patient's problem group is a logical one, taking the student from basics to the advanced aspects of clinical care. 'Core' information about the subject matter relevant to the patient's problem is also summarized, as this information is helpful for answering the questions. The format of the book enables the cases to be used for learning as well as for self-assessment.

In the cases that deal with diagnostic and therapeutic strategies, the student is questioned about the interpretation of all the relevant clinical features presented, in order to compile an array of likely differential diagnoses. They are then asked to identify specific pieces of information in the history and to select an appropriate clinical examination which will narrow down the differential list to the most likely diagnosis. This emphasis is important because, in clinical practice, history and examination alone result in a correct diagnosis in 80–90% of patients. Following this, students are asked to suggest the investigations which would be required to confirm or refute the diagnosis. Once the diagnosis has been reached, students will develop a treatment plan. In general, this plan should first consider conservative non-invasive options (e.g. doing nothing), followed by medical and finally surgical options.

The therapeutic strategy will also have to be conveyed to the patient in a manner that he or she can understand. Therefore in each group, patient problems that will challenge students to develop a counselling strategy have been included. These counselling cases will help students to communicate confidently with patients (one counselling case has been included in the last chapter which gives an idea of the marking system that may be used in an examination situation). This generic learning strategy is followed throughout the book with the aim of reinforcing the skills required to master the problem-solving approach.

J.K. Gupta
G. Mires
K.S. Khan

Abbreviations used for investigations

✓	Investigation required
±	Optional investigation
✗	Investigation not required
βHCG	Beta human chorionic gonadotrophin
BPD	Bi parietal diameter
bpm	Beats per minute
COC	Combined oral contraceptive pill
CT	Computed tomography
CTG	Cardiotocograph
D&C	Dilatation and curettage
FAC	Fetal abdominal circumference
FBC	Full blood count
FHR	Fetal heart rate
FSH	Follicle-stimulating hormone
GnRH	Gonadotrophin releasing hormone
h	Hour
HRT	Hormone replacement therapy
HVS	High vaginal swab
IM	Intramuscular
IV	Intravenous
IVF	*In-vitro* fertilization
IUCD	Intrauterine contraceptive device
L	Litre
LFT	Liver function tests
LH	Luteinizing hormone
min	Minute
MRI	Magnetic resonance imaging
MSU	Midstream specimen of urine
s	Second
SGA	Small for gestational age
STD	Sexually transmitted disease
TFT	Thyroid function tests
TSH	Thyroid-stimulating hormone
U&E	Urea and electrolytes
USS	Ultrasound scan
WCC	White cell count

Part 1

Gynaecology

1 Abnormal Uterine Bleeding

The clinical cases included in this chapter are as follows:
Case 1.1 My periods are regular but heavy
Case 1.2 My periods are heavy and irregular
Case 1.3 I have vaginal bleeding after intercourse

The OSCE counselling cases included in this chapter are as follows:
OSCE counselling case 1.1 Should I have surgery for heavy periods?
OSCE counselling case 1.2 Will hysterectomy affect my sex life?

In order to work through the core clinical cases in this chapter, you will need to understand the following key concepts.

KEY CONCEPTS

Menorrhagia
Excessive loss of blood during menstruation objectively measured to be > 80 mL. In practice, this definition is seldom used and the effect of heavy menstruation on the patient's quality of life is considered to be more important.

Dysfunctional uterine bleeding (DUB)
Menorrhagia not associated with organic disease of the genital tract. It accounts for two-thirds of all menorrhagia cases.
● *Primary* – DUB could be anovular or ovular (common).
● *Secondary* – is due to bleeding disorders such as idiopathic thrombocytopenia, von Willebrand's disease or anticoagulation therapy (uncommon).

Dysmenorrhoea
Painful menstrual periods.
● *Primary* – not associated with organic disease of the genital tract or a psychological cause.
● *Secondary* – a cause can be found (e.g. endometrious, chronic pelvic inflammatory disease).

Premenstrual syndrome
Recurrent *pre*menstrual symptoms (somatic, psychological or behavioural) producing social, family and occupational disturbance, usually relieved by menstruation.

Case 1.1   My periods are regular but heavy

A 34-year-old nulliparous woman presents to the gynaecology out-patient clinic with heavy, regular periods. Her menstrual cycle is 28 days. The periods last for 5 days, with clots during the first 2 days. Up to 40 sanitary towels are required for each period. The patient has no significant dysmenorrhoea, and there is no intermenstrual bleeding. She complains of feeling 'run down' and lacking in energy. Her recent smear was negative, and she is not using any contraception.

Case 1.2   My periods are heavy and irregular

A 47-year-old schoolteacher with two children complains of a 9-month history of heavy irregular periods. Her menstrual cycle is erratic and can vary between 3 and 6 weeks, with periods lasting 5 to 7 days. Prior to the onset of menstrual problems her cycles were regular (every 4 weeks). Her recent cervical smear is negative, and she has no intermenstrual bleeding. The patient has been sterilized.

Case 1.3   I have vaginal bleeding after intercourse

A 29-year-old woman presents with a 4-month history of bleeding after intercourse. She is uncertain about when her last smear was taken. She has four children and currently uses the combined oral contraceptive pill for contraception.

Questions *for each of the case scenarios given*

Q1 What is the likely differential diagnosis?
Q2 What issues in the given history support the diagnosis?
Q3 What additional features in the history would you seek to support a particular diagnosis?
Q4 What clinical examination would you perform and why?
Q5 What investigations would be most helpful and why?
Q6 What treatment options are appropriate?

Case 1.1 My periods are regular but heavy

A1
- Primary dysfunctional uterine bleeding (DUB).
- Uterine leiomyoma (fibroids).
- Uterine endometriosis (adenomyosis).
- Secondary DUB.

A2
Heavy regular periods (menorrhagia) are commonly associated with ovular DUB or fibroids. Anovular DUB would lengthen the cycle and is more common in perimenopausal women (see Case 1.2). Intermenstrual bleeding could be associated with anovular DUB, endometrial or cervical polyp, or carcinoma. Large clots and the large number of sanitary towels required indicate the severity of the problem. Painful periods (dysmenorrhoea) could indicate endometriosis or adenomyosis.

A3
Seek indications of the quality of life (e.g. effect on social life, days off work, etc.) to establish the severity of the problem. Enquire about drug history and family history of bleeding disorders.

A4
Pallor on general examination may indicate anaemia due to blood loss. Bimanual pelvic examination should be undertaken to assess uterine size, mobility and uterine fibroids. Uterine tenderness would indicate a suspicion of adenomyosis.

A5
- **FBC** [✓] To exclude iron deficiency anaemia.
- **TFT** [✗] Not required as a routine investigation.
- **USS** [±] Can give the position, size and number of fibroids or show normal pelvic viscera (DUB).
- **Endometrial biopsy** [✗] Only essential in women over 40 years of age, because in premenopausal women < 40 years, the risk of endometrial cancer is low (1: 100 000). It may be undertaken in younger women with menorrhagia who are not responding to medical treatment.

A6 **SUPPORTIVE**

If investigations are normal, reassure the patient about the absence of pathology. Treat anaemia with iron supplements. Treat primary DUB as described below.

MEDICAL

- Tranexamic acid taken during menses is the treatment of choice. It will reduce menstrual blood loss by approximately 50%.
- Mefenamic acid is useful if there is associated pain. It can be used in conjunction with tranexamic acid.
- Combined oral contraceptive pill.
- Levonorgestrel intrauterine contraceptive device.
- Danazol, but this treatment has side-effects such as acne, weight gain and voice changes.
- *Progestogens are not indicated, and should only be used for anovular DUB, when they should be given in high doses in the second half of the cycle (see Case 1.2).*

SURGICAL

- Not applicable to this patient as her family is *not* complete.
- Endometrial ablation when the family is complete. There are several different types available (e.g. resection, rollerball, laser, hot water, microwave) and they all have a success rate of approximately 80%. Endometrial ablation is not suitable if fibroids are present.
- In cases of fibroids (see Figure 1.1), myomectomy would be suitable if fertility is to be preserved.
- Hysterectomy (abdominal, laparoscopic, subtotal or vaginal) is definitive if the family is complete.

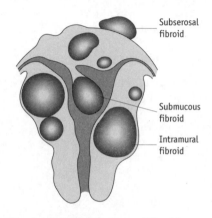

Subserosal fibroid

Submucous fibroid

Intramural fibroid

Figure 1.1 *Different types of fibroids.*

Case 1.2   My periods are heavy and irregular   Answers

A1
- Dysfunctional uterine bleeding (DUB).
- Endometrial pathology (e.g. hyperplasia).
- Climacteric.
- Fibroids/adenomyosis.
- Ovarian pathology.

A2
Perimenopausal women have failing ovarian function and this, associated with an irregularity of the oestrogen/progesterone balance, gives rise to an irregular cycle. In anovular DUB unopposed high oestrogen levels can cause a prolonged cycle in which the endometrium may even undergo hyperplasia (metropathia haemorrhagica – endometrial glands are dilated and crowded). The duration of symptoms is an indication that this condition is unlikely to resolve spontaneously without treatment.

A3
Menopausal symptoms of hot flushes, night sweats, loss of libido and dry skin associated with the climacteric should be sought. Obesity, hypertension and diabetes are risk factors for endometrial cancer and hyperplasia (see Case 4.3).

A4
General examination to exclude pallor. Abdominal examination to exclude pelvic mass secondary to fibroids. Bimanual examination to assess uterine size/mobility and adnexal pathology. This would exclude fibroids and ovarian pathology.

A5
- **FBC** ☑ To exclude iron deficiency anaemia.

- **FSH** ± To check failure of ovarian function if there are any menopausal symptoms. Gonadotrophin levels should be measured during or just after menses.

- **USS** ☑ To exclude uterine and ovarian pathology. Endometrial thickness indicates endometrial pathology. Uterine fibroids or adnexal masses may be visualized.

- **Out-patient hysteroscopy** ☑ To exclude endometrial polyps/submucous fibroids.

- **Out-patient endometrial biopsy** ☑ Endometrial biopsy is the definitive way to exclude hyperplasia and carcinoma of the endometrium. It is recommended that all women over 40 years of age with irregular vaginal bleeding should have an endometrial biopsy. In-patient biopsy (D&C) may be required if out-patient biopsy is inconclusive and ultrasound examination and hysteroscopy are abnormal.

A6   **SUPPORTIVE**

Treat anaemia with iron supplements.

MEDICAL

- If the patient is in the climacteric (perimenopausal), combined hormone replacement therapy may be prescribed (see Case 2.3 and OSCE counselling case 2.1).
- Progestogens in high doses in the second half of the cycle.
- With anovular DUB that has resulted in endometrial hyperplasia (without atypia), progestogen treatment is required in high doses.
- Consider using a levonorgestrel intrauterine device, which has the advantage of releasing continuous progestogens locally in the uterus for up to 5 years.

SURGICAL

- Hysterectomy (abdominal, laparoscopic, subtotal or vaginal) is definitive, particularly when hyperplasia is associated with cellular atypia.

Case 1.3   I have vaginal bleeding after intercourse

A1
- Cervical ectropion.
- Cervical polyp.
- Cervicitis.
- Cervical carcinoma.

A2 The pill is associated with cervical ectropion. (The pill together with pregnancy and puberty as risk factors are commonly remembered as the three Ps).

A3 It would be important to ascertain this woman's social status, her employment, sexual history (age at first intercourse, number of sexual partners) and whether she is a smoker, as all of these are risk factors for a cervical abnormality such as dyskaryosis or carcinoma. A vaginal discharge may be associated with cervicitis.

A4 A careful inspection of the vulva and speculum examination of the vagina and particularly the cervix is mandatory. (See Case 5.1 for details of examination in cases of vaginal discharge).

A5
- **Cervical smear**   ✓   Obtain report of last smear, or take one if there is no bleeding at speculum examination.

- **Vaginal or cervical swabs for microscopy and culture**   ±   Only if infection is suspected, or in cases associated with vaginal discharge.

- **Colposcopy and cervical biopsies**   ±   Mandatory if there is any suspicion of malignancy, or if cervical smear result is abnormal.

A6 **SUPPORTIVE**

- Reassure the patient if there is no pathology.

MEDICAL

- Infection should be treated with appropriate antibiotics according to the results of culture and sensitivity reports.

SURGICAL

- If a polyp is evident, this should be avulsed and sent for histopathological assessment. This can be done as an out-patient procedure without anaesthesia.
- Cervical ablation – if the smear is normal, a cervical ectropion can be reasonably treated in the out-patient clinic (e.g. with cryotherapy, cold coagulation, laser, or large loop excision of the transformation zone – LLETZ).

OSCE counselling case 1.1 Should I have surgery for heavy periods?

A 45-year-old woman presents with an 18-month history of increasingly heavy periods. She has a regular cycle with 7 days of bleeding every 28–30 days. Clinical examination and investigations are unremarkable. A diagnosis of DUB is reached.

Q1 If she opted for surgical management, what factors would you consider important when counselling her?

OSCE counselling case 1.2 Will hysterectomy affect my sex life?

A 44-year-old woman is having considerable problems with menorrhagia (DUB), which have been unresponsive to medical treatment. She has been offered a hysterectomy by her gynaecologist, who has given her some time to consider this option. She mentioned this to a friend, who told her that the operation 'ruins your sex life and makes you incontinent'.

Q1 Can you reassure her? What factors would you consider important when counselling her?

OSCE counselling case 1.1   Should I have surgery for heavy periods?

Answers

A1   The surgical approaches that are available (i.e. endometrial ablation or hysterectomy).

- If a hysterectomy is decided upon, consideration would need to be given to the route (i.e. vaginal/abdominal or laparoscopically assisted and, if abdominal, whether this would be total or subtotal). In addition, consideration would need to be given to whether the ovaries should be removed in order to reduce the risk of ovarian cancer. If so, then HRT would be necessary to protect against cardiovascular disease and osteoporosis. Ovaries may be conserved to continue functioning until the natural menopause.
- If endometrial ablation is decided upon, the patient would need to be advised that amenorrhoea is not guaranteed, and that there is a possibility that hysterectomy may be required at the time of surgery if a complication arises, or at a later date if the ablation is not successful. In addition, pregnancy should be avoided and sterilization may be considered at the same time as ablation.
- For either procedure, consideration needs to be given to detailing the surgical procedure, the need for an anaesthetic, the duration of stay in hospital, the need for convalescence and time off work, and the loss of fertility.

OSCE counselling case 1.2   Will hysterectomy affect my sex life?   **Answers**

A1
- *Bladder function* – the bladder innervation may be altered, but evidence of an increased incidence of incontinence is conflicting.
- *Bowel function* – again there is conflicting evidence, with some studies suggesting an increase in the incidence of irritable bowel syndrome and constipation, and others showing no change.
- *Sexual function* – both psychological and physical factors influence sexual function. It is generally accepted that sexual function remains unchanged and may even improve.

The patient should be reassured about these aspects, particularly in view of the benefits she is expected to derive from the operation in terms of symptomatic relief from menorrhagia.

2 Amenorrhoea and menopause

The clinical cases included in this chapter are as follows:
Case 2.1 My periods are infrequent. I have not had any for 7 months
Case 2.2 I have intolerable menstrual periods
Case 2.3 Should I take HRT?

The OSCE counselling case included in this chapter is as follows:
OSCE counselling case 2.1 HRT compliance

In order to work through the core clinical cases in this chapter, you will need to understand the following key concepts.

KEY CONCEPTS

Puberty
Time of onset of ovulatory and endocrine ovarian function making an individual capable of reproduction.

Delayed puberty
Lack of secondary sexual characteristics by the age of 14 years, or primary amenorrhoea.

Amenorrhoea
Lack of menstruation (it is a symptom, not a diagnosis).
- *Primary* – lack of menstruation by 16 years of age in a girl with normal growth and secondary sexual characteristics.
- *Secondary* – amenorrhoea for 6 months or for a duration of more than three times the length of previous menstrual cycles after an individual has formerly had menstrual periods.

Oligomenorrhoea
Infrequent periods with a menstrual cycle longer than 35 days.

Menopause
Lack of menstruation for more than 12 months associated with cessation of ovarian function and reproductive capacity.

Premature menopause
Menopause before the age of 35 years.

Hirsutism
Excessive growth of sexual (androgen-dependent) hairs.

Virilism
Androgenic changes more extensive than hirsutism, including amenorrhoea, breast atrophy, clitoromegaly and temporal balding.

Case 2.1   My periods are infrequent. I have not had any for 7 months

A 24-year-old woman attends a gynaecology clinic concerned that she has not had a menstrual period for 7 months. She had her first period when she was 12 years old. Her periods have been gradually becoming more infrequent. She keeps athletically fit, and has recently been training for a marathon and has lost some weight. She has a normal healthy appetite and diet. She claims not to have been sexually active for the past 12 months. Her home pregnancy test is negative.

Case 2.2   I have intolerable menstrual periods

A 35-year-old woman has been experiencing pelvic pain, irritability, bloatedness and breast pain for 3 to 4 days before her periods. These symptoms have occurred cyclically over a period of 4 to 6 months, and they disappear following the onset of menses. Her periods are regular and painful but not heavy. She has two children and uses condoms for contraception. There is no history of psychiatric illness.

Case 2.3   Should I take HRT?

A slim 52-year-old university lecturer presents with an 18-month history of amenorrhoea and a three-year history of hot flushes and night sweats. She has a family history of heart disease and breast cancer.

Questions *for each of the case scenarios given*

Q1   What is the likely differential diagnosis?
Q2   What issues in the given history support the diagnosis?
Q3   What additional features in the history would you seek to support a particular diagnosis?
Q4   What clinical examination would you perform and why?
Q5   What investigations would be most helpful and why?
Q6   What treatment options are appropriate?

Case 2.1 My periods are infrequent. I have not had any for 7 months

A1
- Secondary amenorrhoea:
    stress-related amenorrhoea;
    polycystic ovarian syndrome (PCOS);
    hyperprolactinaemia;
    hyper/hypothyroidism.
- Premature menopause.

A2 Pregnancy, the commonest cause of secondary amenorrhoea, is unlikely in this case as the patient is not sexually active and a urinary pregnancy test is negative. Although she normally keeps fit, the excessive recent training over and above her normal routine level of fitness is likely to be a possible cause of her amenorrhoea. Moreover, as she has a normal diet, she does not have anorexia nervosa-related amenorrhoea.

A3 An additional history should be obtained about menopausal symptoms (i.e. hot flushes, night sweats), in order to exclude premature menopause. Precise information about weight loss will be helpful, as sudden excessive loss of >10 kg is associated with amenorrhoea. PCOS would normally be associated with infertility and oligomenorrhoea. Headaches and visual disturbances may suggest optic chiasma pressure from a prolactinoma in the anterior pituitary. Symptoms of intolerance of extremes of temperature, feeling very energetic or lethargic, and excessive weight loss or weight gain would be consistent with hyper/hypothyroidism. A drug history (e.g. progestogens and major tranquillizers such as phenothiazines) should be obtained, as the use of certain drugs is associated with lack of menstruation.

A4 The patient's weight should be measured (this may not be diagnostic, but it will be helpful in management and follow-up). The condition of the skin and hair may indicate thyroid abnormalities. Hirsutism and acne are associated with PCOS. Evidence of striae and stigmata of virilization may be an indication of severe PCOS or a hormone-producing tumour. A breast examination should be performed to ensure normality of secondary sexual characteristics and to check for galactorrhoea (a sign of prolactinoma). The visual fields should be examined in cases of prolactinoma. An abdomino-pelvic mass would indicate a possible pregnancy or hormone-producing ovarian tumour.

A5
- **Pregnancy test** ☑ Hospital pregnancy tests are more reliable than home tests.

- **LH and FSH** ☑ An LH:FSH ratio of 3:1 would indicate PCOS. An FSH level of > 25 IU/mL would be associated with premature menopause.

- **Serum prolactin** ☑ If hyperprolactinaemia is confirmed, further tests (CT or MRI of head for pituitary adenoma, and visual field assessment) for prolactinoma may be required.

- **USS** ± A pelvic ultrasound examination may reveal small peripheral cysts in polycystic ovaries. Thick endometrium is associated with polycystic ovaries, but thin endometrium is associated with premature menopause.

- **TFT** ✗ This test is only required in cases with symptoms or signs of hypo- or hyperthyroidism, or if there is hyperprolactinaemia which is known to be associated with hypothyroidism.

A6 SUPPORTIVE

After cessation of excessive training and an increase in body weight, spontaneous resolution and return of menses would be expected.

MEDICAL

- PCOS – combined oral contraceptive (COC) if the patient wishes to have periods. If pregnancy is desired, then commence ovulation induction (see Case 6.2).

- Menopause – COC, combined hormone replacement therapy (HRT) (see Case 2.3 and OSCE counselling case 2.1).

- Hyperprolactinaemia – bromocriptine, cabergoline (dopamine agonists).

SURGERY

- Prolactinomas – rarely required nowadays.

- PCOS – ovarian drilling.

Box 2.1 *Additional considerations in cases of primary amenorrhoea*

- Developmental disorder of uterus or genital outflow tract
  Imperforate hymen/transverse vaginal septum
  Vaginal/uterine atresia
- Chromosomal disorder
  Turner's syndrome
- Anorexia nervosa

Case 2.2   I have intolerable menstrual periods

A1
- Premenstrual syndrome (PMS).
- Secondary dysmenorrhoea:
  endometriosis – adenomyosis;
  pelvic inflammatory disease.
- Pelvic venous congestion.

A2
PMS is common around the age of 35 years. This complex problem of unknown aetiology occurs during the week before menstruation, and is classically resolved by menstruation. Adenomyosis is associated with painful periods that are usually heavy.

A3
Tension, aggression, depression and 'fluid' retention are other common symptoms of PMS. Any susceptibility to accidents, criminal acts and suicide indicates severe disability, which occurs in 3% of cases.

A4
General examination with pelvic examination is necessary to exclude 'organic' disease (e.g. pouch of Douglas nodularity, which may be due to endometriosis). A mental state examination is essential, as depression and neurosis can present as PMS.

A5
- **Symptom diary**   ✓   The diagnosis of PMS is confirmed by establishing that the recurrent symptoms are the same, that they occur regularly, and that there is a symptom-free period between menses.

- **USS**   ±   A pelvic ultrasound examination may show ovarian endometrioma (termed *chocolate cysts*).

- **Diagnostic laparoscopy**   ±   Not required as a routine test, but may be considered if there is any suggestion of an organic cause for the pelvic pain.

A6   **SUPPORTIVE**

- Treatment is empirical because the cause is unknown. Sympathetic handling, support, reassurance about the absence of pathology, and understanding (particularly by family members) are very important.
- Cognitive and relaxation therapy.
- Any treatment has a high rate (75%) of placebo response.

MEDICAL

- COC (not progesterone alone).
- Evening primrose oil.
- Vitamin B_6 (pyridoxine).
- Selective serotonin reuptake inhibitors (SSRIs) are effective in severe cases.
- High-dose oestrogens may be helpful, but progestogens would be required as well to prevent endometrial hyperplasia/malignancy.
- GnRH agonists can be used to stop ovarian function temporarily. Symptomatic relief is both diagnostic and therapeutic.
- Diuretics are not usually successful.

SURGICAL

- A last-resort solution would be bilateral oophorectomy. Total abdominal hysterectomy and bilateral salpingo-oophorectomy would represent a permanent solution. 'Oestrogen-alone' HRT as a non-cyclical preparation could be used subsequently without causing a recurrence of symptoms.

Case 2.3 Should I take HRT? Answers

A1 Menopause.

A2 The average age of menopause in the UK is 51 years. This patient has been suffering from menopausal symptoms for 3 years, indicating that the climacteric and menopause are occurring at the appropriate age.

A3 Other symptoms of the menopause include depression, loss of libido, hair loss, dry skin, and painful intercourse due to dry vagina (dyspareunia). It is important to check whether there is any family history of osteoporosis, breast cancer or ischaemic heart disease, and early menopause, as well as checking factors such as smoking, previous Colles' or hip fracture, sedentary lifestyle and low body mass index. It would be important to exclude any evidence of vaginal bleeding, which would warrant further investigations (see Case 4.3).

A4 General examination, including blood pressure measurement is necessary to exclude hypertension. Examination of the breasts is mandatory, but it is likely that if the patient is registered with a general practice, she would have been called for breast screening through a national screening programme at the age of 51 years. Pelvic examination would only be necessary if a recent cervical smear had not been taken.

A5 The diagnosis of menopause is firm in this case, and therefore a determination of FSH levels is not required. However, it may be prudent to offer this patient genetic counselling and screening for breast cancer (*BRAC1* and *BRAC2* genes) if at least two first-degree relatives (mother or sisters) have been affected by breast cancer.

A4 This patient would need careful counselling about the benefits and disadvantages of hormone replacement therapy (HRT), as she has a family history of heart disease and breast cancer. A heart disease history should encourage the use of HRT, whereas a history of breast cancer would suggest that it should be used with caution, although HRT would not be contraindicated if the patient was adequately counselled (see below). Counselling should be reinforced with written literature.

A6 There are several different preparations of HRT available (oral preparations, patches, implants and a gel). The oral types have stronger cardiovascular protective effects as they have a greater influence on the modification of lipid profiles (increasing HDL and lowering LDL levels) due to the first-pass metabolism effect.

This patient should be given *combined* oestrogen and progestogen preparations, as she has an intact uterus. 'Oestrogen-only' preparations would be suitable for a hysterectomized patient.

The effects of the different preparations range from monthly withdrawal bleeding to three-monthly withdrawal bleeding or no withdrawal bleeding. The latter *continuous* combined preparations would be highly suitable for this patient, as she has been amenorrhoeic for at least one year. This would improve her long-term compliance with HRT.

OSCE counselling case 2.1   HRT compliance

A 48-year-old woman has menopausal symptoms. As a result of this and the fact that she has a family history of osteoporosis, she wishes to start hormone replacement therapy (HRT). However, compliance is a problem in women who start HRT.

Q1   What issues should be considered for improving this woman's compliance?

Q2   What would be an appropriate screening programme for this patient if she was happy to start HRT?

OSCE counselling case 2.1 HRT compliance

 • Explore any concerns that she may have about the treatment.
- Ensure that she has realistic expectations of the treatment.
- Emphasize the benefits of treatment – both short-term symptomatic benefits (e.g. relief from flushes) and long-term benefits (e.g. cardioprotective effects).
- Provide accurate information about the risks and potential complications (e.g. cancer and thromboembolism).
- Discuss the appropriate method of administration and type of HRT for the patient.
- Ensure regular review.
- Give the patient a leaflet/literature about HRT.

Box 2.2 *Benefits and disadvantages of HRT*

Benefits

1. Reduces risks of:
   - fractures, osteoporosis – more so in slim individuals with a sedentary lifestyle;
   - cardiovascular disease (i.e. coronary artery disease, stroke);
   - Alzheimer's disease;
   - dental disease;
   - ovarian cancer;
   - endometrial cancer;
   - colon cancer.

2. Improves:
   - mood;
   - energy;
   - dry skin;
   - hair loss;
   - insomnia;
   - sensory urgency.

Disadvantages

Oestrogenic side-effects	*Progestogenic side-effects*
Breast tenderness	Breast pain
Nipple sensitivity	Fluid retention
Vaginal discharge	Bloating
Leg cramps	Increased appetite

Breast cancer risk
- Background risk – 45 per 1000 women.
- 5 years of HRT use – 47 per 1000 women (i.e. 2 per 1000 increased risk).
- 10 years of HRT use – 52 per 1000 women (i.e. 7 per 1000 increased risk).

This small increase in breast cancer risk is associated with a more favourable prognosis following treatment than in those who have breast cancer without HRT.

- Pre-treatment:
  blood pressure measurement;
  weight;
  breast examination;
  cervical smear;
  pelvic examination.

- Six-monthly:
  weight;
  blood pressure measurement.

- Yearly:
  breast examination.

- Three-yearly:
  mammography;
  cervical smear;
  pelvic examination.

3 Incontinence and prolapse

The clinical cases included in this chapter are as follows:
Case 3.1   Every time I cough, I leak urine
Case 3.2   I have to rush to the toilet otherwise I leak urine
Case 3.3   I feel something coming down

The OSCE counselling cases included in this chapter are as follows:
OSCE counselling case 3.1   What investigations am I going to have for leaking urine?
OSCE counselling case 3.2   Can my prolapse be treated without surgery?

In order to work through the core clinical cases in this chapter, you will need to understand the following key concepts.

KEY CONCEPTS

Continence
Ability to hold urine in the bladder at all times except when voiding.

Incontinence
Involuntary urine loss which is objectively demonstrable and which is a social or hygienic problem.

Genuine stress incontinence (synonymous with sphincter incompetence)
Involuntary urine loss associated with stress due to increased intra-abdominal pressure (e.g. while coughing, exercising, etc.), but in the absence of bladder muscle (detrusor) contractions.

Detrusor instability
Involuntary urine loss associated with loss of inhibition of detrusor contractions during stress.

Frequency
Normal frequency is usually every 4 h, and it decreases by 1 h per decade. Voiding more often than six times a day or more frequently than every 2 h is usually regarded as abnormal.

Nocturia
Interruption of sleep due to micturition more than once every night. Voiding twice at night over the age of 70 years and three times over the age of 80 years is considered to be within normal limits.

Uterovaginal prolapse
Descent of the pelvic genital organs towards or through the vaginal introitus:
- *first-degree* – descent of the cervix and uterus but not up to the introitus;
- *second-degree* – descent of the cervix up to the introitus;
- *third-degree* – descent of the cervix and the whole uterus through the introitus;
- Procidentia – whole of the uterus out of the introitus.

Case 3.1   Every time I cough, I leak urine

A 36-year-old parous woman complains of involuntary urinary loss on exercise, sneezing or coughing. She has suffered from this problem since the birth of her first child 10 years ago, which was assisted with forceps. She is fit and healthy, but has to wear sanitary protection all the time. Otherwise she voids 5 or 6 times a day and once at night, passing good volumes of urine without difficulty.

Case 3.2   I have to rush to the toilet, otherwise I leak urine

A 60-year-old woman complains of voiding difficulties. She has a frequency of 10–12 times during the day. At night she gets up 3 or 4 times to void. There is also involuntary urinary loss, particularly when she cannot reach the toilet immediately. She has suffered from this problem for the last 20 years, but it has gradually been worsening since her periods stopped 10 years ago. She is not on hormone replacement therapy. Recently the urinary loss has increased so much that it has become a major hygienic problem. Her social activities have become severely restricted because of the worsening of the condition. She has been treated for urinary tract infections on several occasions in the past. There is no history of diabetes or hypertension.

Case 3.3   I feel something coming down

A 56-year-old shopkeeper presents to a gynaecology clinic with a 3-month history of a sensation of 'something coming down'. She feels a 'lump' in her vagina, which is worse towards the end of the day, in association with a dragging backache. She has had four vaginal deliveries, one of which was assisted by forceps. There were no macrosomic babies. She does not have urinary or bowel incontinence.

Questions *for each of the case scenarios given*

- **Q1** What is the likely differential diagnosis?
- **Q2** What issues in the given history support the diagnosis?
- **Q3** What additional features in the history would you seek to support a particular diagnosis?
- **Q4** What clinical examination would you perform and why?
- **Q5** What investigations would be most helpful and why?
- **Q6** What treatment options are appropriate?

A1
- Sphincter incompetence (genuine stress incontinence or GSI).
- Detrusor instability (urge incontinence).
- Mixed incontinence (GSI and detrusor instability).
- Neurological disorder (uncommon).

A2
A history of involuntary urinary loss due to a rise in intra-abdominal pressure (e.g. during exercise, sneezing or coughing) in the absence of voiding difficulties is suggestive but not a definite feature of sphincter incompetence. Difficult childbirth can be a risk factor. Quality of life is measured by the impact of the urinary problem on the patient's usual activities.

A3
A specific history of urgency and urge incontinence with or without associated urinary tract infections is suggestive of detrusor instability. In this condition, urinary frequency is far more than 5 or 6 times per day, and sleep is also frequently disturbed due to nocturnal frequency. Sphincter incompetence will often be associated with multiparity, prolonged labour, and symptoms of uterovaginal prolapse and faecal incontinence. In neurological disorders such as multiple sclerosis, incontinence will usually be a secondary symptom.

A4
Physical examination should be performed with a comfortably full bladder, when incontinence should be demonstrated by asking the patient to cough. However, this finding does not conclusively indicate GSI. Pelvic examination is usually normal in women with incontinence. Incontinence is sometimes associated with pelvic masses (e.g. a large fibroid uterus causing pressure effects). Occasionally, incontinence is associated with neurological disease. Sphincter incompetence may be associated with evidence of perineal deficiency on inspection and uterovaginal descent on straining.

A5
It is important not to rely solely on the patient's history and examination for diagnosis.

- **MSU** ☑ To exclude urinary tract infection.

- **Urodynamic** ☑ To differentiate between sphincter incompetence and detrusor instability. In
  investigations sphincter incompetence urodynamics are normal. That is:

  urine flow rate is > 15 mL/s;

  bladder capacity is >300 mL;

  residual volume is < 50 mL;

  bladder pressure rises by < 15 cmH$_2$O during filling;

  detrusor remains stable throughout filling and voiding.

A6

SUPPORTIVE

The local incontinence advisory service should be involved in management. Sphincter incompetence can be treated conservatively using techniques for pelvic floor re-education (pelvic floor exercises and other physiotherapy techniques, including vaginal cones, perineometry, electrical stimulation, etc.).

MEDICAL

Drug therapy includes alpha agonists (e.g. phenylpropanolamine) which increase urethral resistance.

SURGICAL

Surgery is used to support the proximal urethra. This is commonly achieved by elevation of the bladder neck using colposuspension. Alternative surgical techniques include slings and para-urethral injection of Teflon. These techniques should be employed in preference to anterior colporrhaphy or anterior repair, which do not have as long-term a benefit as colposuspension procedures.

A1
- Detrusor instability (urge incontinence).
- Sphincter incompetence (genuine stress incontinence – GSI).
- Mixed incontinence (GSI and detrusor instability).
- Neurological disorder (uncommon).

A2
A history of urgency, frequency and nocturia with or without associated urinary tract infections is highly suggestive of detrusor instability. At this patient's age, a frequency of every 2 h is abnormal. Quality of life is measured by the patient's social activities being restricted and her having hygienic problems. Postmenopausal atrophic changes of the bladder will also be a contributory factor in this case.

A3
Fluid intake habits, particularly in relation to tea, coffee and alcohol, are important with regard to the symptomatology. Haematuria may indicate a bladder stone or tumour. Involuntary urinary loss due to a rise in intra-abdominal pressure (e.g. caused by exercise, sneezing or coughing) in the absence of voiding difficulties is suggestive of sphincter incompetence (GSI). Incontinence may be associated with symptoms of uterovaginal prolapse and faecal incontinence. In neurological disorders such as multiple sclerosis, incontinence will usually be a secondary symptom.

A4
Physical examination should be performed with a comfortably full bladder, when incontinence may be demonstrated by asking the patient to cough. Signs of oestrogen deficiency may be evident on inspection of the genitalia. There may be uterovaginal descent on straining. Pelvic examination may reveal a pelvic mass – which may be the cause of urinary symptoms due to pressure effects. Occasionally incontinence is associated with neurological disease. Examination of S2, 3 and 4 dermatomes is essential.

A5
- **MSU**   ☑   To exclude urinary tract infection.

- **Urodynamic**   ☑   To differentiate between sphincter incompetence and detrusor instability. In
  investigations   detrusor instability, urodynamics might show:

   reduced bladder capacity (< 300 mL);

   high bladder pressure, increasing to > 15 cmH$_2$O during filling;

   spontaneous detrusor contractions during filling, or contractions in response to provocation such as a change in posture.

   Urodynamic investigations are not essential as a matter of routine. They should, however, be undertaken in patients who are not responding to supportive and medical therapeutic measures.

A6   **SUPPORTIVE**

The incontinence advisory service should be involved in management. Fluid intake habits may have to be altered in order to manage the symptoms (e.g. last drink at 18.00 hours, reducing tea, coffee and alcohol intake). Detrusor instability can be treated conservatively using techniques for bladder training to re-establish central bladder control.

MEDICAL

Drug therapy in this case might include hormone replacement therapy. Urinary tract infections should be treated with appropriate antibiotics. Anticholinergic drugs may produce detrusor relaxation (side-effects include dry mouth, blurred vision and constipation).

SURGICAL

There is no place for surgery as a primary intervention. Only when all other methods have been exhausted should complex procedures such as Clam's cytoplasty be considered. These are end-stage procedures with a high morbidity rate and long-term problems.

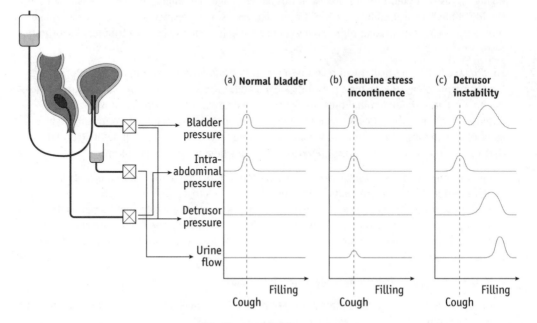

(a) **Normal bladder**

- No increase in detrusor pressure with filling
- No detrusor contraction with cough
- No urine flow with cough

(b) **Genuine stress incontinence**

- No increase in detrusor pressure with filling
- No detrusor contraction with cough
- Urine flow with cough

(c) **Detrusor instability**

- Detrusor contraction after cough
- Urine flow with detrusor contraction if increase in bladder pressure is sufficient to overcome urethral pressure

Figure 3.1 *Urodynamic investigations.*

Case 3.3   I feel something coming down   Answers

A1
- Cystocele.
- Uterine prolapse:
    primary;
    secondary;
    tertiary
        (procidentia).
- Rectocele.
- (Enterocele – pouch of Douglas hernia which contains loops of bowel.)

A2 'Something coming down' is a symptom of the various types of uterovaginal prolapse. Prolapse in the premenopause is uncommon. Childbirth and particularly traumatic delivery indicates that there may have been possible pelvic floor damage. It is difficult to ascertain the type of prolapse from the history alone without examination. It is said that women who have a physically demanding job are at high risk of prolapse. The sensation of prolapse is typically worst at the end of the day.

A3 It is important to ascertain a history of urinary incontinence (see Cases 3.1 and 3.2). In general, stress incontinence is not associated with cystocele. Constipation or difficulty in emptying fully can suggest a rectocele. The use of HRT may reduce the risk of prolapse. Postnatal exercises are considered to be a preventative measure for future prolapse. Smoking history and cough associated with smoking or respiratory illnesses may exacerbate the symptoms of prolapse. Chronic cough is also a poor prognostic factor for the success of prolapse surgery. It is also important to establish whether the patient is sexually active.

A4 Record the patient's weight and perform a general physical examination to assess her fitness for operation if this is intended. Exclude an abdominal mass, and examine the external genitalia to assess signs of atrophy. Ask the patient to cough in order to detect any stress incontinence (although elicitation of this at the time of examination is not conclusive evidence of her incontinence). During straining, any components of prolapse can be described, but the different types can only be distinguished using a Sim's speculum in the left lateral position. A bimanual examination should be performed to exclude a pelvic mass.

A5 The diagnosis is primarily made on the basis of the clinical examination. If there is concurrent incontinence, then urodynamics would be mandatory prior to surgery (see OSCE counselling case 3.1).

A6 **SUPPORTIVE**
- Weight control.
- Stop smoking.
- Pelvic floor exercises.
- Vaginal pessaries (e.g. ring or shelf) may be used to provide symptom relief if the patient is unfit for operation, or if she wishes to avoid surgery. Pessaries are more likely to be helpful in women with a prominent suprapubic arch and strong perineal body for support, otherwise the pessary is easily expelled. Pessaries are generally replaced every 4 to 6 months.

MEDICAL

Vaginal oestrogen cream or HRT.

SURGICAL

- *Cystocele* – anterior repair (colporrhaphy) – or colposuspension. The latter should be the preferred option if there is urodynamically established concurrent genuine stress incontinence.
- *Uterovaginal prolapse* – cervical amputation with shortening of the uterosacral ligaments (Manchester–Fothergill repair). This operation should only be performed if a vaginal hysterectomy is not possible.
- *Vaginal hysterectomy* – this removes the prolapsed organ. Anterior repair and posterior repair are performed if appropriate. The vaginal vault should be suspended.
- *Rectocele* – posterior repair and perineal repair in cases where there is a deficient perineum from previous childbirth (posterior colpoperineorrhaphy).

In all of these surgical interventions, the rate of recurrence is high if preventative measures (e.g. HRT, reduction in body weight, and stopping smoking in the case of chronic cough) are not implemented. In any repair operation, the vagina and introitus should not be obliterated, in order to prevent dyspareunia or inhibition of intercourse.

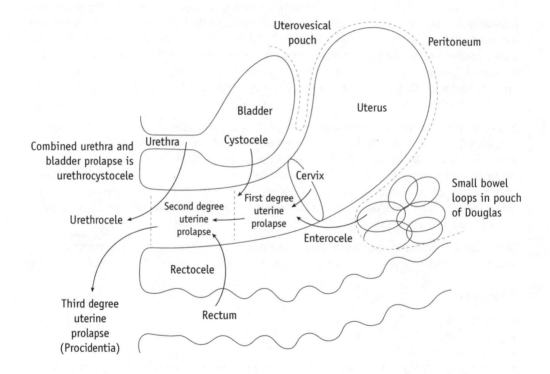

Figure 3.2 *Different types of prolapse.*

OSCE counselling case 3.1   What investigations am I going to have for leaking urine?

A 56-year-old woman presents with a history of incontinence of urine and urinary frequency. She describes a sudden urge to pass urine followed by incontinence, but she can also leak when lifting and coughing. You have excluded a urinary tract infection, and pelvic examination is unremarkable. You decide to perform urodynamic investigations.

Q1 In counselling this patient, what points would you wish to make about the reasons for performing the investigation?

Q2 What does the investigation involve?

OSCE counselling case 3.2   Can my prolapse be treated without surgery?

A 65-year-old woman is referred with a procidentia that is reducible. There are no pelvic masses or urinary or faecal problems.

Q1 Discuss the non-surgical management options and any potential problems that may be encountered with these treatments, as the patient is medically unfit for surgery.

OSCE counselling case 3.1 What investigations am I going to have for leaking urine?

A1
- The investigation measures the pressure in the bladder and how the bladder works when it is filled and emptied.

- The performance of the test will identify why the woman's incontinence is occurring (i.e. whether it is due to a weakness in the supports of the bladder, or whether it occurs because the bladder is sensitive and contracts with very little urine in it).

- It is important to differentiate between the two, because the treatment for each problem is different (i.e. surgical options for sphincter incompetence and medical options for detrusor instability). Surgical treatment for detrusor instability could make the patient's problem worse.

- The procedure is performed in the out-patient clinic.

A2
- A catheter is placed in the patient's bladder and in her back passage (rectum).

- Each is connected to a machine which measures pressure.

- The bladder is filled through the catheter in the bladder, and the pressure in the bladder is measured while this is being done. The amount of fluid present in the patient's bladder before she feels that she needs to pass water will be measured.

- She will sit on a commode while this is being done in case she cannot control her bladder.

- She will then be asked to stand up and cough, to see whether urine leaks.

- Finally, she will be asked to empty her bladder into the commode so that the flow rate can be measured.

- Some minor discomfort may be experienced when the catheters are inserted.

- The patient will be followed up in the clinic after the results of the test have been obtained.

OSCE counselling case 3.2   Can my prolapse be treated without surgery?

A1   *Management options*

- No treatment, and just reassurance if the patient remains problem-free. The procidentia is unlikely to cause any serious harm, but it is considered to be a progressive condition.

- Topical weekly/twice weekly oestrogen application in the vagina to counteract excoriation and dryness. Alternatively, combined HRT can be prescribed.

- To help to keep the procidentia reduced, insert a ring pessary of appropriate size.

- If the ring pessary fails to stay in place, a shelf pessary of appropriate size should be tried. This has a higher likelihood of success, but is incompatible with sexual function.

Problems

- Ring and shelf pessaries will require replacement every 6 months. They can cause bleeding due to pressure on atrophic vaginal skin. If excoriation or ulceration occur, the pessaries should be left out and topical oestrogen cream should be prescribed daily for 2 to 4 weeks.

- Sometimes the pessaries can cause urinary retention and/or faecal impaction.

4 Neoplasia

The clinical cases included in this chapter are as follows:
Case 4.1 My cervical smear is abnormal
Case 4.2 I am menopausal and my abdomen is distending
Case 4.3 I have gone through the change and I have recently had some vaginal bleeding

The OSCE counselling cases included in this chapter are as follows:
OSCE counselling case 4.1 My smear report is unsatisfactory. Do I have cancer?
OSCE counselling case 4.2 I have warts. Will I get cancer?

Case 4.1   My cervical smear is abnormal

A 35-year-old single woman is found to have an abnormal smear on routine screening. She has had regular smears since the age of 25 years, and previous smears have been normal. She has two children aged 2 and 7 years. She is separated from her partner, who fathered both children. She is currently using the oral contraceptive pill, and she does not have a stable relationship.

Case 4.2   I am menopausal and my abdomen is distending

A 68-year-old woman presents with gradual enlargement of the abdomen, changes in bowel habit and weight loss. The general practitioner had felt a lower abdominal mass and referred the patient urgently to the gynaecology clinic.

Case 4.3   I have gone through the change and I have recently had some vaginal bleeding

A 54-year-old woman has been amenorrhoeic for the past 18 months, and recently started to have some vaginal bleeding. Her last cervical smear, taken 2 years ago, was normal. She is not on HRT.

Questions *for each of the case scenarios given*

Q1 What is the likely differential diagnosis?
Q2 What issues in the given history support the diagnosis?
Q3 What additional features in the history would you seek to support a particular diagnosis?
Q4 What clinical examination would you perform and why?
Q5 What investigations would be most helpful and why?
Q6 What treatment options are appropriate?

Case 4.1 My cervical smear is abnormal Answers

A1 Abnormal smear could be associated with:
- infection or inflammation;
- dyskaryosis (which may be reflective of cervical intra-epithelial neoplasia);
- malignancy.

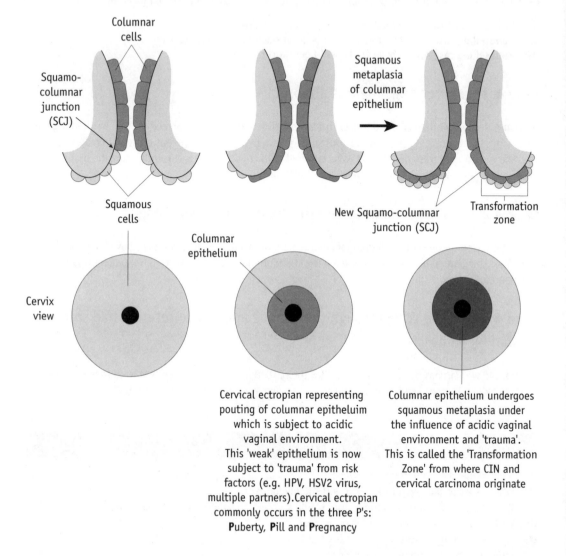

Figure 4.1 *Mechanisms of abnormal smears. HPV,* human papilloma virus; *HSV,* herpes simplex virus.

A2 Although an abnormal smear often leads to concern about cancer, in the majority of cases it is associated with a benign condition (infection, inflammation or cervical intra-epithelial neoplasia). From the given history, one can only elicit some of the risk factors for cervical intra-epithelial neoplasia (e.g. multiparity and multiple sexual partners). However, it is not possible to be certain of the diagnosis without further investigation.

A3 The history of additional risk factors associated with cervical intra-epithelial neoplasia and cancer should be obtained (e.g. young age at first intercourse, sexually transmitted disease (particularly HPV and HSV-2), cigarette smoking and low socio-economic status. Gynaecological symptoms such as inter-menstrual bleeding and post-coital bleeding may be indicative of a local lesion. Vaginal discharge may be associated with infection or inflammation. The current partner's history of sexually transmitted disease may be relevant.

A4 Inspection of the vulva and vagina may reveal discharge or infection. Inspection of the cervix may show a cervical eversion, a polyp or a tumour. In most cases, however, cervical inspection with the naked eye will be normal. Bimanual examination should be performed to assess cervical mass, cervical fixity, pelvic mass and pelvic tenderness. In the case of cervical cancer, examination will also determine staging, but this is usually performed under anaesthesia together with cystoscopy. If a sexually transmitted disease is diagnosed, the male partner will also need to be examined.

A5
- **Colposcopy and cervical biopsies** ☑ If the abnormality in the smear shows moderate or severe dyskaryosis, colposcopy (inspection of the cervix under magnification using a binocular microscope) should be performed. At colposcopy, directed biopsies should be taken to establish a histological diagnosis.

- **Cervical and vaginal swabs** ± If infection is suspected, appropriate vaginal and cervical swabs should be obtained for microbiological investigation.

A6 **SUPPORTIVE**

Explanation depending on findings of clinical examination and degree of abnormality of smear report and need for further investigation and follow-up. The specific treatment depends on the cause.

MEDICAL

Infection – treat according to cause and repeat the smear after six months.

SURGICAL

- *Cervical ectropion* – observation only, or cryotherapy for symptomatic relief.
- *Cervical intra-epithelial neoplasia* – excision or ablation of the lesion and follow-up smears.
- *Cervical cancer* – chest X-ray, intravenous pyelogram, cystoscopy, examination under anaesthetic, cervical biopsy, surgery and/or radiotherapy according to stage.

Table 4.1 *Appropriate actions to be taken in response to cervical smear report*

Cervical smear report	Appropriate action
Normal	Repeat smear every 3 years
Inflammation	Test for and treat any infections
	Repeat smear at 6 months – if abnormality is persistent refer for colposcopy
Mild dyskaryosis	Repeat smear at 6 months – if abnormality is persistent refer for colposcopy
Moderate/severe dyskaryosis	Refer for colposcopy
Glandular cells	Cone biopsy, hysteroscopy

Case 4.2 I am menopausal and my abdomen is distending Answers

A1
- Pelvic mass arising from the ovary, Fallopian tube or uterus.
- Ascites.
- Bladder distension.
- Bowel problems (e.g flatus, faeces, cancer).

A2 Gradual abdominal distension and changes in bowel habits in a postmenopausal patient with a pelvic mass are highly suspicious of an ovarian tumour.

A3 Nulliparity, early menarche, late menopause, higher social class and history of breast cancer are associated with ovarian neoplasm. Use of the oral contraceptive pill has a protective effect. Postmenopausal bleeding can be a symptom of ovarian cancer, but it may also be due to endometrial or Fallopian tube cancer. A urinary and bowel history should be obtained. The diagnosis cannot be established without further investigation.

A4 A general examination should be performed, looking for lymphadenopathy and lower limb oedema. Chest examination should specifically exclude pleural effusion. Ascites should be demonstrated on abdominal examination. Ascites is dull to percussion in the flanks, compared to central dullness in an ovarian cyst. Bimanual examination will detect pelvic mass, its relationship to the uterus and its mobility.

A5 *Investigations should be performed to exclude ovarian tumour.*

- **CA 125** ✓ This is an ovarian tumour marker.

- **USS** ✓ Abdomino-pelvic ultrasound examination can demonstrate the presence of ascites. If a mass is detected, its nature (whether cystic or solid) and origin may be determined by the scan.

- **Chest X-ray** ✓ This may be required in order to assess pleural effusion, or as a pre-operative test for fitness for anaesthesia.

- **Ascitic sample** ± This may be taken for cytological examination.

A6 **SUPPORTIVE**

Pain relief, and drainage of ascites or effusions.

SURGICAL

Surgical excision of tumour (hysterectomy, bilateral salpingo-oophorectomy, omentectomy and debulking of tumour, aiming to reduce it to < 2 cm in diameter).

MEDICAL

Chemotherapy depending on the stage determined at surgery.

Case 4.3 I have gone through the change and I have recently had some vaginal bleeding

A1
- Atrophic vaginitis.
- Endometrial polyp, hyperplasia and carcinoma.
- Cervical polyp and cancer.
- Adnexal malignancy (uncommon).

A2 This vaginal bleeding is classified as postmenopausal bleeding (PMB), with a 10–15% likelihood of endometrial pathology, particularly cancer.

A3 Post-coital bleeding could also suggest a cervical polyp or cancer. Hypertension, diabetes and obesity are risk factors for endometrial hyperplasia and cancer. Information about cervical smear reports must be obtained, bearing in mind that a negative smear history does not exclude the possibility of cervical cancer in women with symptoms of postmenopausal bleeding. Symptoms of hot flushes and night sweats indicate that the HRT dose may not have been sufficient. In this case there might also be a history of painful dry vagina during intercourse, which would suggest atrophic vaginitis.

A4 A general examination should be performed to exclude pallor and lymphadenopathy. Speculum examination will demonstrate local causes such as atrophic vaginitis and cervical polyps or carcinoma. Bimanual examination should be performed to assess uterine size, mobility and adnexal pathology.

A5 *The primary aim of investigations is to exclude gynaecological cancer.*

- **Out-patient endometrial biopsy** ✓ It is mandatory to obtain an endometrial sample for histological assessment to exclude hyperplasia or cancer.

- **USS** ✓ A pelvic ultrasound examination is performed for endometrial thickness measurement and adnexal masses (ovarian tumours can present as PMB). Current evidence suggests that an endometrial thickness of < 4 mm reduces the likelihood of endometrial cancer substantially.

- **Out-patient hysteroscopy** ✓ This allows direct visualization of the uterine cavity, which is particularly useful for excluding endometrial polyps.

- **In-patient (D&C)** ± This is only required if the out-patient assessment is either inadequate or impossible to perform.

A6 **SUPPORTIVE**

No pathology is found in the majority of cases. If this is so after thorough investigations, then the patient can be reassured.

MEDICAL

- Vaginal oestrogen cream would supplement the existing HRT for treatment of atrophic vaginitis. Alternatively, the HRT dose may be altered to provide a preparation with a higher oestrogen content.
- Progestogens for simple endometrial hyperplasia without cellular atypia.

SURGICAL

- Polypectomy.
- Total hysterectomy and bilateral salpingo-oophorectomy for complex endometrial hyperplasia, particularly with associated atypia.
- If endometrial cancer or another gynaecological cancer is found, it is treated according to stage.

OSCE counselling case 4.1   My smear report is unsatisfactory. Do I have cancer?

Having had a routine cervical smear 2 weeks earlier, a 36-year-old woman returns to see you (her GP) about the result. She has received a card through the post indicating that the smear was 'unsatisfactory', and she is very anxious about the implications of this.

The smear result, which you have available, is as follows:

- good cellularity;
- endocervical cells present;
- moderate dyskaryosis.

Q1 Counsel this patient about her smear result.

OSCE counselling case 4.2   I have warts. Will I get cancer?

A 26-year-old woman presents with genital warts. She is worried that the virus that causes warts also causes cervical cancer. She has never had a cervical smear.

Q1 What would you say to her?

OSCE counselling case 4.1   My smear report is unsatisfactory. Do I have cancer?   Answers

 A1   The nature of the report:
  does not indicate cancer;
  indicates that abnormal cells are present;
  requires further investigation to exclude pathology. The pathology is usually a precancerous condition;
  suggests that if a precancerous condition is found, it will require further treatment to prevent progression.

The nature of the investigation and treatment would be as follows:
  referral for colposcopy (examination of the cervix with magnifying binoculars);
  the need for punch biopsies or large loop excision of the transformation zone (LLETZ);
  treatment by laser/cold coagulation/LLETZ.

Regular follow-up smears would be needed according to the findings.

OSCE counselling case 4.2   I have warts. Will I get cancer?   Answers

A1
- Many factors are associated with the development of cervical cancer, and the virus that causes warts is just one of them.
- Wart virus is very common, and there are many different types. Not all of these types are associated with cervical cancer.
- Even if the warts are caused by a type of virus that is associated with cervical cancer, the risk of developing it is small.
- Regular cervical smears will identify cervical change prior to the development of cervical cancer. These changes are easily cured before they become cancerous.
- Perform a speculum examination (to confirm that the cervix appears normal) and take a cervical smear. A cervical smear should be taken every 3 years.

5 Discharge and pain

The clinical cases included in this chapter are as follows:
Case 5.1   I have constant irritating vaginal discharge
Case 5.2   I am unwell and have abdominal pain and discharge
Case 5.3   My periods are painful and I also have pain during intercourse

The OSCE counselling cases included in this chapter are as follows:
OSCE counselling case 5.1   I am having a diagnostic laparoscopy. Should I be concerned?
OSCE counselling case 5.2   I have had a diagnostic laparoscopy. What happens next?

In order to work through the core clinical cases in this chapter, you will need to understand the following key concepts.

Key Concepts

Pelvic inflammatory disease (PID)
Infection of the upper genital tract, with salpingitis as the most prominent feature.
● *Primary PID* – due to infection ascending from the lower genital tract.
● *Secondary PID* – due to direct spread from adjacent organs (e.g. appendix).

Sexually transmitted disease (STD)
Genital tract infection due to sexually transmitted infective organisms (e.g. gonorrhoea, chlamydia, herpes, etc.). PID is a serious complication of STD.

Chronic pelvic pain
Constant or intermittent, cyclic or acyclic pain located in the pelvis, which may or may not be related to menstruation, is associated with adverse effects on quality of life, and has lasted for more than 6 months. No pelvic pathology is found in 50–60% cases with chronic pelvic pain.

Dysmenorrhoea
Pain associated with menstruation.
● *Primary dysmenorrhoea* – pain not associated with any organic disease. It is common at menarche.
● *Secondary dysmenorrhoea* – pain associated with organic disease such as endometriosis or PID.

Dyspareunia
Pain associated with sexual intercourse. This can be classified as superficial or deep dyspareunia.

Case 5.1   I have constant irritating vaginal discharge

A 25-year-old single woman has vulval and vaginal itching and discharge. Her recent cervical smear was normal. She has recently started a new relationship and is currently using the oral contraceptive pill. There are no urinary symptoms. She recently had a severe bout of flu for which she was given antibiotics.

Case 5.2   I am unwell and have abdominal pain and discharge

A 22-year-old woman presents with fever, lower abdominal and pelvic pain and a foul-smelling vaginal discharge. Her last menstrual period was 1 week ago. She has recently changed her sexual partner. There are no urinary or bowel symptoms.

Case 5.3   My periods are painful and I also have pain during intercourse

A 30-year-old nulliparous professional woman presents with severe and incapacitating menstrual pain that requires bed-rest and interferes with her employment. The menstrual pain has been present for 1 year, but it has gradually been increasing in severity over the last few months. The patient's periods are not heavy, and she has no desire for fertility. She recently started a relationship and finds intercourse very painful. The couple has been using condoms for contraception.

Questions *for each of the case scenarios given*

Q1   What is the likely differential diagnosis?
Q2   What issues in the given history support the diagnosis?
Q3   What additional features in the history would you seek to support a particular diagnosis?
Q4   What clinical examination would you perform and why?
Q5   What investigations would be most helpful and why?
Q6   What treatment options are appropriate?

Case 5.1 | I have constant irritating vaginal discharge

A1
- Infection:
  Candida;
  trichomonas vaginalis;
  bacterial vaginosis;
  chlamydia;
  gonorrhoea;
  herpes.
- Inflammation.
- Foreign body (e.g. forgotten tampon).
- No pathology (e.g. cervical ectropion).

A2
Associated itching, a new sexual partner, use of the oral contraceptive pill and broad-spectrum antibiotics could all be associated with Candida infection (although most infections involve a mixture of organisms). Urinary symptoms, absent in this case, could be associated with chlamydia, gonorrhoea or herpes.

A3
Specific inquiry should be directed towards the colour and consistency of the discharge. Typically, a thin green discharge is associated with bacterial vaginosis, a thick white discharge is due to *Candida*, a grey frothy discharge is due to *Trichomonas* and a yellow mucopurulent discharge is due to chlamydia or *Gonococcus*. The relationship between discharge and menstruation should be established. *Candida* is usually premenstrual and *Gonococcus* is postmenstrual. Intense itching that is worse at night is a feature of *Candida*, but could be associated with *Trichomonas*. Pain, dyspareunia and burning are features of *Trichomonas* and gonococcal infection. Poor personal hygiene, and the use of talcum powder, deodorants, douches and tight synthetic undergarments may lead to itching. The history of sexually transmitted disease in the woman's partner should also be obtained. A family history of diabetes and symptoms of polyuria and polydipsia may indicate diabetes mellitus, which is associated with *Candida* infections.

A4
Inspection of the vulva may reveal erythema or congestion, which is much more marked with *Candida* than with *Trichomonas*. The erythema may extend perianally. Gonococcal infection may be associated with painful vulval swelling and uretheral discharge. Multiple small vesicles with ulcers are associated with herpes. Speculum examination may demonstrate discharge with associated erythema. A search should be made for any foreign bodies (e.g. a forgotten tampon). A sample of the discharge should be taken for microscopy, culture and sensitivity. *Trichomonas* is associated with reddish-purple spots in the vagina and cervix (strawberry cervix). Cervical ectropion may be a cause of discharge without infection. A bimanual examination should be performed to assess pelvic tenderness, which may suggest pelvic inflammatory disease. The male partner should also be examined.

A5
- **Urine dipstick** ☑ For glycosuria.

- **MSU** ☑ For microscopy and culture.

- **pH of discharge** ☑ The pH of the discharge is alkaline (> 5) in *Trichomonas* infections or bacterial vaginosis.

- **Whiff test of discharge** ☑ If the discharge is mixed with potassium hydroxide, it produces a fishy odour in bacterial vaginosis.

- **Microscopy of discharge** ✓ A sample of the discharge should be mixed with saline and examined under the microscope. No organisms are usually seen in physiological discharge. Mycelial filaments and spores are seen in *Candida* infection. Motile flagellated protozoa may be seen in *Trichomonas* infection.

- **Gram stain of discharge** ✓ Gram staining of the discharge will show blue cells with a serrated border in bacterial vaginosis, and Gram-negative diplococci in *Gonococcus* infection.

- **Vaginal and cervical swabs** ✓ Depending on the patients' risk factors for sexually transmitted disease and the findings at examination, swabs should be obtained from the upper vagina, endocervix and urethra for culture. Separate swabs should be taken for chlamydia. Investigations of the male partner should also be carried out.

A6 SUPPORTIVE

Advice on personal hygiene and clothing. Specific treatment depends on the cause.

MEDICAL

- No organisms – no treatment if the problem is not persistent. Otherwise treat as *Candida* infection.

- Candida – clotrimazole cream or oral flucanozole.

- Trichomonas or bacterial vaginosis – metronidazole.

- Chlamydia – doxycycline.

- Gonococcus – penicillin, erythromycin.

- Herpes – acyclovir.

- Treat the male partner simultaneously.

SURGICAL

Cervical ectropion – observation only, or cryotherapy for symptomatic relief.

Case 5.2 I am unwell and have abdominal pain and discharge

Answers

A1
- Acute pelvic inflammatory disease:
  - sexually transmitted disease;
  - iatrogenic cause (e.g. due to intrauterine contraceptive device);
  - secondary PID.
- Acute abdomen:
  - ectopic pregnancy;
  - ovarian cyst;
  - conditions related to bowel.

A2
Pyrexia, pelvic pain and foul-smelling vaginal discharge are very probably due to pelvic inflammatory disease. A recent change of sexual partner is a risk factor for pelvic inflammatory disease. Although ectopic pregnancy is unlikely, due to the fact that this patient's last menstrual period was just 1 week ago, menstrual history is an unreliable indicator of pregnancy.

A3
Specific inquiry should be directed towards the nature and onset of the pain, and the pattern of fever. Swinging pyrexia is typically associated with a pelvic abscess. A sexual history should be obtained, enquiring about the number of sexual partners, any recent casual sexual encounters, history of sexually transmitted disease, and previous history of pelvic inflammatory disease. The oral contraceptive pill reduces the risk of pelvic inflammatory disease, but does not necessarily prevent it. Copper intrauterine contraceptive devices are associated with PID, and the latter is also associated with recent gynaecological surgery and delivery or miscarriage.

A4
General examination should include measurement of temperature, blood pressure and pulse to assess shock. Inspection of the vulva, vagina and cervix may demonstrate discharge with associated erythema. A sample of the discharge should be taken for microbiology. Separate swabs for *Gonococcus* and chlamydia should be taken from the endocervix and urethra. Digital examination of the cervix may show excitation. Bimanual examination should be performed to assess pelvic tenderness, which may suggest pelvic inflammatory disease. It may also reveal a mass, which could be a pelvic abscess.

A5

• **Urine HCG**	✓	To exclude pregnancy.
• **FBC**	✓	A full blood count should be taken for leucocytosis.
• **U&E**	±	Urea and electrolytes are required for any renal effects if sepsis is suspected.
• **USS**	✓	A pelvic ultrasound examination should be performed to support clinical examination, particularly examining any pelvic masses (e.g. ovarian cyst).
• **MSU**	✓	For microscopy and culture.
• **Vaginal and cervical swabs**	✓	Samples of the discharge should be examined under the microscope, with Gram staining and culture.
• **Blood cultures**	±	These are necessary if there are signs of septicaemia.

A6 **SUPPORTIVE**

If there is clinical shock, resuscitation should be performed while examination and investigations are being undertaken. An indwelling catheter should be used to monitor urine output.

MEDICAL

Oxygen, fluid resuscitation and intravenous broad-spectrum antibiotics should be administered in cases of septic shock. Otherwise, treat PID with antibiotics directed at the suspected organism or according to culture and sensitivity reports.

SURGICAL

Once the patient is relatively stable then, depending on the diagnosis, surgery may be required:

- PID with pelvic mass that is not responding to medical treatment – surgical drainage of abscess;

- acute abdomen – laparotomy.

Case 5.3 My periods are painful and I also have pain during intercourse

A1
- Endometriosis.
- Chronic pelvic inflammatory disease.
- No associated pathology (primary dysmenorrhoea).

A2 The patient's age would argue against the diagnosis of primary dysmenorrhoea, which usually occurs in teenage girls. The combination of painful intercourse (dyspareunia) and painful periods is typical of endometriosis, a condition that is more prevalent in nulliparous women of high social class.

A3 Pelvic pain due to endometriosis typically starts several days before the period and remains severe in intensity for several days after it. However, primary dysmenorrhoea usually eases within 1 to 2 days after the onset of menses. Previous infertility and a family history of the condition may support the possibility of endometriosis. Occasionally endometriosis is associated with bowel or bladder symptoms, including haematuria or rectal bleeding during periods.

A4 Speculum examination may reveal spots of endometriosis in the vagina, particularly in the posterior fornix. Bimanual examination should be performed to assess uterine fixity and pelvic tenderness, which might suggest either pelvic inflammatory disease or endometriosis. Nodularity in the uterosacral ligaments is typical of endometriosis. There may be an adnexal mass associated with endometrioma.

A5
- **Investigations for gynaecological infections** ✓ Investigations should be performed for infection if the history and examination suggest pelvic inflammatory disease (see Case 5.2).

- **USS** ✓ A pelvic ultrasound scan should be performed which, although not specific for endometriosis, might reveal ovarian endometrioma.

- **Diagnostic laparoscopy** ✓ The definitive diagnosis of endometriosis is established by laparoscopy. No pathology is seen at laparoscopy in 50–60% of patients with chronic pelvic pain.

A6 **SUPPORTIVE**

- Explain the nature of the problem. Endometriosis is not a curable disease.

- Monitor the disease and its symptoms by means of ultrasound scan or MRI scan.

MEDICAL

- The aim of medical treatment is to provide pain relief and induce amenorrhoea.

- Non-steroidal anti-inflammatory drugs (NSAIDS) may be given for dysmenorrhoea.

- The combined oral contraceptive pill (given continuously for at least 3 months).

- Progestogen (oral or injectable).

- Danazol (side-effects include acne, hirsutism, voice changes and weight gain).

- GnRH analogues (side-effects include menopausal symptoms that are treatable with HRT).

- Endometriosis (and its symptoms) often recur after the cessation of medical treatment.

SURGICAL

Specific treatment of symptomatic endometriosis depends on the severity of the condition and the patient's desire for fertility.

- Mild endometriosis (few peritoneal spots at laparoscopy, no scarring):
surgical ablation or excision, possibly followed by medical treatment for 3 to 6 months (if fertility is not desired).

- Moderate endometriosis (peritoneal and ovarian spots at laparoscopy, minor scarring):
surgical ablation or excision plus adhesiolysis, possibly followed by medical treatment for 6 months.

- Severe endometriosis (peritoneal and ovarian spots at laparoscopy, severe scarring, tubal block):
surgical excision of endometriosis (hysterectomy and oophorectomy if appropriate); medical treatment for 6 months as for moderate endometriosis after conservative surgery.

OSCE counselling case 5.1 I am having a diagnostic laparoscopy. Should I be concerned?

A patient with chronic pelvic pain is going to be admitted to hospital for diagnostic laparoscopy under general anaesthetic. Her clinical pelvic examination and pelvic ultrasound scan are normal.

Q1 What information will you need to provide when counselling her about the investigation?

OSCE counselling case 5.2 I have had a diagnostic laparoscopy. What happens next?

The above patient underwent an uneventful diagnostic laparoscopy. The laparoscopic findings of a normal pelvis are shown in the diagram.

Q1 What information will you need to provide when counselling her prior to discharge from hospital?

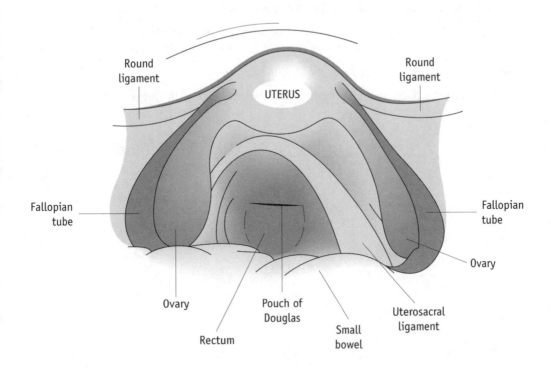

Figure 5.1 *Laparoscopic findings.*

OSCE counselling case 5.1 I am having a diagnostic laparoscopy. Should I be concerned?

- Laparoscopy is being performed to look for a cause for the pelvic pain. It allows a telescopic examination of the gynaecological and abdominal organs. It is regarded as a minor operative procedure and is performed as a day case, but it does carry risks.

- The procedure is conducted as follows. Once the patient is asleep under general anaesthetic, air is introduced into their abdomen by a small needle inserted in the navel. This enables a telescope to be inserted via a small incision in the navel. The surgeon will then examine the pelvic area and reproductive organs to see if there is any obvious reason for the pelvic pain, such as endometriosis or pelvic adhesions. If this is the case, these conditions may be treated surgically there and then if appropriate. If there is no obvious cause for the pain, no further treatment is necessary. The surgery does not usually result in any noticeable discomfort, and the patient can be discharged home a few hours after laparoscopy. There are two or three cuts on the abdomen which are approximately half a centimetre long, and may not even require stitches. If stitches are required, they may be self-absorbing so may not need to be removed later. There should be minimal scarring from these incisions under normal circumstances.

- Although laparoscopy is a relatively safe procedure, like any other surgical procedure it is not without risks and side-effects. These include possible damage to organs inside the abdomen. However, the likelihood of such complications occurring is minimal.

- If complications do occur, they may have to be dealt with there and then with an open operation. If this is the case, an in-patient stay for several days post-operatively may be required.

- There are also risks associated with the anaesthetic.

- A written leaflet about diagnostic laparoscopy should be given to the patient.

OSCE counselling case 5.2   I have had a diagnostic laparoscopy. What happens next?

A1
- The laparoscopy shows a completely normal pelvis. This is the case in 50–60% of women who undergo laparoscopy for chronic pelvic pain.

- It is reassuring in that there is no evidence of endometriosis, adhesions, pelvic inflammatory disease or other gynaecological pathology.

- This does not exclude other causes of pelvic pain (e.g. irritable bowel syndrome).

- In the absence of organic pathology, no specific gynaecological treatment is required. However, further investigation of other possible causes of pain might have to be performed.

- If the two or three cuts on the abdomen have been stitched, provide information about how they are to be managed. Also provide information about simple post-operative painkillers, and reassure the patient that scarring from these incisions will be minimal under normal circumstances.

- Following discharge from hospital, if the postoperative pain does not show progressive improvement, the patient must contact the hospital.

- Advise the patient about follow-up arrangements. If the pelvic pain does not settle in response to simple measures, assessment in a combined pain clinic (where an assessment can be made by a psychologist or anaesthetist interested in chronic pain management) may be necessary.

- Provide the patient with a written leaflet.

6   Infertility

The clinical cases included in this chapter are as follows:
- **Case 6.1**   We are unable to have a pregnancy
- **Case 6.2**   My periods are irregular and I cannot conceive
- **Case 6.3**   I have been pregnant before, but I cannot conceive now

The OSCE counselling cases included in this chapter are as follows:
- **OSCE counselling case 6.1**   Is my coital timing correct?
- **OSCE counselling case 6.2**   Should my ovaries be stimulated to produce eggs?

In order to work through the core clinical cases in this chapter, you will need to understand the following key concepts.

Key Concepts

Infertility (subfertility)
Involuntary failure to conceive despite 12 months of unprotected sexual intercourse (it is a symptom, not a diagnosis).
- *Primary infertility* – no previous pregnancy.
- *Secondary infertility* – previous pregnancy (regardless of outcome).

Causes of infertility

Male factor	25%
Anovulation	25%
Unexplained	25%
Tubal blockage and other causes	25%

(tubal blockage is more common when there is a high prevalence of pelvic infection)

Case 6.1   We are unable to have a pregnancy

A young couple present with a history of inability to conceive despite unprotected intercourse for the past 2 years. The couple have had no previous conceptions. The gynaecological history is unremarkable. The female partner has had regular menstrual cycles without the oral contraceptive pill. The frequency of intercourse is two to three times per week. In addition, the couple have been timing intercourse according to an ovulation kit for the last 6 months. There is a history of mumps in childhood in the male partner.

Case 6.2   My periods are irregular and I cannot conceive

A 28-year-old woman presents with an inability to conceive despite unprotected intercourse for 18 months. Her periods are erratic, sometimes with 6 weeks between periods. She started taking the pill at the age of 18 years and stopped 18 months ago. Her periods were irregular prior to commencement of the pill. She has had no previous pregnancies, but her partner has fathered a child previously.

Case 6.3   I have been pregnant before, but I cannot conceive now

A 32-year-old married nurse presents with an 18-month history of inability to conceive following removal of an intrauterine contraceptive device (IUCD). The IUCD had been in place for 3 years, was inserted after the birth of her second child, and was removed because of her wish to try for another child. Her periods are regular with mild dysmenorrhoea, and she is with the same partner who fathered her previous children.

Questions *for each of the case scenarios given*

Q1   What is the likely differential diagnosis?
Q2   What issues in the given history support the diagnosis?
Q3   What additional features in the history would you seek to support a particular diagnosis?
Q4   What clinical examination would you perform and why?
Q5   What investigations would be most helpful and why?
Q6   What treatment options are appropriate?

Case 6.1 We are unable to have a pregnancy Answers

A1
- Primary infertility:
   male factor;
   tubal block;
   anovulation;
   unexplained infertility.

A2
Regular periods are usually a feature of an ovulatory menstrual cycle. The couple have been timing intercourse according to an ovulation kit, and it should be confirmed that intercourse is occurring before ovulation. It is unlikely that the cause of the problem is anovulation. Although none of the above factors can be confirmed or excluded from the given history alone, the history of mumps supports the possibility that male factor is the cause.

A2
A diagnosis of tubal block is supported by a gynaecological history of vaginal discharge associated with pelvic pain. Pelvic pain may also be due to endometriosis, which could be associated with tubal blockage. Male factor may also be associated with primary infertility, so information should be sought about general health, testicular descent, urethral discharge (e.g associated with sexually transmitted disease) and occupational exposure (e.g. excess heat, smoking, alcohol and drugs).

A2
Obesity and hirsutism on general examination may indicate polycystic ovarian syndrome. The breasts should be examined for galactorrhoea. Speculum examination might reveal discharge or infection. Bimanual examination should be performed to assess uterine fixity and pelvic tenderness, which might suggest either pelvic inflammatory disease or endometriosis. The male partner should also be examined, looking for signs of virilization, gynaecomastia, cryptorchidism, varicoceles, testicular size, and epididymal and prostatic tenderness.

A5
- **Semen analysis** ✓ This should be performed on a fresh specimen after 3 day's abstinence. Any abnormality of semen should be confirmed on three specimens obtained at monthly intervals. In the case of low sperm count and/or motility, additional investigations should include microbiological tests for infection, such as chlamydia, and an immunological test for antisperm antibodies. Sperm abnormalities should be investigated and managed by a specialist. Karyotype and hormonal assays (FSH, LH and testosterone) may be indicated as part of the investigation for oligo/azoospermia.

- **Mid-luteal serum progesterone** ✓ This confirms ovulation.

- **Chlamydia** ✓ To rule out asymptomatic infection.

- **USS** ± Depending on the history and examination of the female partner, a pelvic ultrasound scan may be indicated to look for polycystic ovaries.

- **Laparoscopy and dye hydrotubation and/or hysterosalpino-gography** ± If there is a possibility of pelvic adhesions due to a history of infection, endometriosis or positive chlamydia, then these tests may be performed to assess the severity of the condition and its amenability to treatment.

- **Rubella IgG** ✓ To confirm the female partner's immunity to rubella. If she is non-immune, rubella immunization (and appropriate contraception) is necessary.

A6 *Female partner* – folic acid supplements to prevent neural-tube defects.

Male partner – specific treatment of male factor (oligo/azoospermia) depends on the cause.

MEDICAL

- Infection – treat according to cause, or empirically for chlamydia.
- Hypogonadotrophic hypogonadism – clomiphene citrate or gonadotrophins.

SURGICAL

- Varicocele – high ligation of varicocele.
- Obstruction of vas – vasovasostomy.
- Consider assisted conception.
- Donor insemination.
- Intrauterine insemination of prepared partner's sperm.
- *In-vitro* fertilization and embryo transfer (IVF-ET).
- Intracytoplasmic sperm injection (ICSI).

Case 6.2 My periods are irregular and I cannot conceive

Answers

A1
- Primary infertility:
  anovulation (polycystic ovaries, prolactinaemia);
  unexplained infertility.

A2 A diagnosis of anovulation is supported by a history of menstrual irregularity that also pre-dates the use of the oral contraceptive pill.

A3 A recent history of weight changes and hirsutism should be noted. A history of galactorrhoea would indicate hyperprolactinaemia. A past history of sexually transmitted disease and a family history of polycystic ovaries should be sought.

A4 Obesity and hirsutism on general examination may indicate polycystic ovarian syndrome. The breasts should be examined for galactorrhoea. A speculum and bimanual examination should be performed. The male partner should also be examined.

A5
- **Mid-luteal serum progesterone** ✓ Confirmation of anovulation is essential. As the menstrual cycle is irregular, the test should be taken weekly and the results interpreted in the light of the date of the next menstrual period.

- **LH and FSH** ✓ In polycystic ovarian syndrome, the LH/FSH ratio is > 2.

- **Serum prolactin** ✓ To test for hyperprolactinaemia. If confirmed, further tests (CT or MRI of head for pituitary adenoma, and visual field assessment) for prolactinoma may be required.

- **TFT** ✗ Not required as a routine test. It is only necessary in hyperprolactinaemia which may be associated with hypothyroidism.

- **Semen analysis** ✓ To rule out male factor.

- **Chlamydia** ✓ To rule out asymptomatic infection.

- **USS** ± A pelvic ultrasound scan to assess for polycystic ovaries.

- **Laparoscopy and dye hydrotubation and/or hysteroscalpingography** ± If there is a possibility of pelvic adhesions due to a history of infection, endometriosis or positive chlamydia, then these tests may be performed to assess the severity of the condition and its amenability to treatment. These tests may also be indicated if infertility persists despite treatment.

- **Rubella IgG** ✓ To confirm the female partner's immunity to rubella. If she is non-immune, rubella immunization (and appropriate contraception) is necessary.

A6 *Female partner* – considering a diagnosis of anovulation:

- folic acid supplements to reduce the risk of neural-tube defects;

- timing intercourse around ovulation (using an ovulation kit if necessary);

- induce ovulation with clomiphene citrate (see OSCE 6.2).

Specific treatment depends on the cause.

MEDICAL

- polycystic ovarian syndrome – induce ovulation. If clomiphene is not successful, use gonadotrophins.

- Hyperprolactinaemia – bromocriptine.

SURGICAL

- Polycystic ovarian syndrome – ovarian drilling.

- *In-vitro* fertilization and embryo transfer (IVF-ET) – a last-resort treatment.

Case 6.3 I have been pregnant before, but I cannot conceive now Answers

A1
- Secondary infertility:
  tubal blockage;
  unexplained infertility.

A2
The IUCD may have been associated with a clinical or subclinical infection that has led to damage of the Fallopian tubes. Regular periods are usually a feature of ovulation, and previous pregnancies from the same partner indicate that male factor may not be involved. These factors would have to be investigated.

A3
A diagnosis of tubal block due to pelvic infection will be supported by an obstetric history of deliveries associated with postpartum pyrexia and foul lochia, or by a gynaecological history of vaginal discharge associated with pelvic pain. Pelvic pain may also be due to endometriosis, which could be associated with tubal blockage. Male factor may also be associated with secondary infertility, so information about the frequency and timing of intercourse should be sought.

A4
Speculum examination might demonstrate discharge or infection. Bimanual examination should be performed to assess uterine fixity and pelvic tenderness, which might suggest either pelvic inflammatory disease or endometriosis. The male partner should also be examined for testicular size and varicocele (see Case 6.1).

A5
- **Laparoscopy and dye hydrotubation and/or hysterosalpingography** ✓ To assess for tubal blockage, severity of the condition and its amenability to treatment.

- **Mid-luteal serum progesterone** ✓ Confirmation of anovulation is essential.

- **Semen analysis** ✓ To rule out male factor.

- **Chlamydia** ✓ To rule out pelvic infection.

- **USS** ± A pelvic ultrasound scan may be indicated on the basis of abnormal pelvic examination.

- **Rubella IgG** ✓ To confirm the female partner's immunity to rubella. If she is non-immune, rubella immunization (and appropriate contraception) is necessary.

A6
Female partner – folic acid supplements to prevent neural-tube defects. Specific treatment depends on the cause.

MEDICAL

- Pelvic infection – treat according to cause or empirically for chlamydia.

- Endometriosis – medical treatment (this leads to anovulation).

SURGICAL

- Endometriosis – for mild endometriosis, ablation or excision at laparoscopy improves fertility and obviates the need for medical treatment.

- Tubal block – adhesionolysis, salpingostomy, and excision of blocked segment and re-anastomosis.
- Assisted conception (*in-vitro* fertilization and embryo transfer) is an alternative.

OSCE counselling case 6.1   Is my coital timing correct?

A 30-year-old woman has been trying for her first pregnancy for 10 months. She thought that pregnancy occurs around the time of menstruation, but has recently heard from a friend that this is not the case. She feels that she does not understand the best time for her to conceive. She has always had a regular 32-day cycle.

Q1 How would you counsel this patient about coital timing?

OSCE counselling case 6.2   Should my ovaries be stimulated to produce eggs?

A 28-year-old woman attends for the results of her infertility investigations. These are summarized in the table below.

Test	Value obtained	Normal range
Luteal phase progesterones	7 ng/mL, 12 ng/mL and 9 ng/mL on three separate occasions	> 20 ng/mL
Prolactin	300 IU/mL	150–500 IU/L
LH	12 mIU/mL	1.8–13.4 mIU/mL
FSH	4 mIU/mL	3.0–12.0 mIU/mL
Rubella	Immune	—
Husband's semen	Normal	—

Q1 What is the potential reason for this patient's infertility, and what first-line treatment are you going to recommend for rectifying this?

OSCE counselling case 6.1 Is my coital timing correct?

A1
- Conception occurs around the time of ovulation, not during menses.

- Ovulation occurs 14 days prior to the onset of menstruation. Therefore a 32-day cycle means that ovulation occurs on day 18 (32–14).

- Sperm can survive for up to 4 days.

- Eggs can only survive for 24 h.

- Intercourse should *occur* before ovulation, so that there are sperm ready to fertilize the egg.

- The 'fertile period' therefore lasts for 5 days (i.e. days 14–19 counted from the first day of menstruation in a 32-day cycle). However, ovulation can occur slightly early or slightly late in different cycles, and it would be reasonable to regard the fertility period as occurring 1 week around the expected time of ovulation.

- Abstinence is not beneficial. As long as intercourse occurs every 36–48 h during the fertile period, sperm will be in the vicinity of the egg at around the time of ovulation.

- The likelihood of pregnancy in any one cycle is 15–25% (not 100%), even in a perfectly normal (fertile) couple having intercourse at the right time.

OSCE counselling case 6.2 Should my ovaries be stimulated to produce eggs?

A1
- The three luteal phase progesterones are low, indicating that anovulation is the most likely cause of infertility. The LH/FSH ratio is consistent with the diagnosis of polycystic ovaries.

- The first-line therapy for ovulation induction is clomiphene citrate.

- The starting dose is 50 mg per day from day 2–6 of the patient's menstrual cycle. A luteal-phase progesterone level should be checked in order to evaluate the response to treatment. Intercourse should be timed, using a home ovulation kit if necessary.

- If there is no response to treatment, the dose of clomiphene citrate can be increased by 50 mg in the subsequent cycle, going up to a maximum of 150 mg per day.

- Treatment should be for a maximum of 6 ovulatory months. This usually leads to ovulation, but pregnancy is only achieved in 50% of cases. Pregnancy loss occurs in about 20% of cases, so it cannot be guaranteed that the mother will take home a baby even if pregnancy is achieved.

- The risks of clomiphene treatment are multiple pregnancy (5% risk) with associated poor pregnancy outcome, and hyperstimulation of the ovaries (rare). There is an association with ovarian cancer, and prolonged use is therefore inadvisable.

- If clomiphene treatment is unsuccessful, ovulation may be induced with injectable treatment (gonadotrophins), and assisted conception techniques may be required. However, adoption, fostering and child-free life are other alternatives.

7 Fertility control

The clinical cases included in this chapter are as follows:
Case 7.1 I had unprotected intercourse last night and wish for contraception
Case 7.2 My family is complete and I now wish to be sterilized
Case 7.3 I am pregnant and don't want to be
Case 7.4 I have just had a baby and I now require contraception

The OSCE counselling cases included in this chapter are as follows:
OSCE counselling case 7.1 How should I take 'morning after' pills?
OSCE counselling case 7.2 How should I take the pill?

Case 7.1 I had unprotected intercourse last night and wish for contraception

A 32-year-old woman has unprotected intercourse during mid-cycle and comes to the family planning clinic seeking advice for contraception. She is also in need of reliable long-term contraception, as she wishes to delay her family for at least 3 years. She smokes 10 cigarettes a day.

Case 7.2 My family is complete and I now wish to be sterilized

A 27-year-old woman with three children requests sterilization. She has three sons aged 7 years, 5 years and 3 years. She has been using the oral contraceptive pill since her last child was born. She has recently separated from her husband after a 10-year marriage, and she feels that she does not want to have any more children. She does not currently have a sexual partner.

Case 7.3 I am pregnant and don't want to be

A 22-year-old woman finds out that she is pregnant. She is not in a stable relationship and she requests termination of pregnancy. She was using condoms for contraception, and she has not had any previous pregnancies.

Case 7.4 I have just had a baby and I now require contraception

A 38-year-old woman had a normal delivery 14 days ago and is fully breastfeeding without supplementation. This is her second child, and the two pregnancies were narrowly spaced. She previously became pregnant within 2 months of using the progesterone-only pill. She now wishes to have good contraception.

Questions for each of the case scenarios given

Q1 What issues in the given history have implications for the request?
Q2 What additional features in the history would you seek to support her request?
Q3 What clinical examination would you perform and why?
Q4 What investigations would be most helpful?
Q5 What treatment options are available?

Case 7.1 I have had unprotected intercourse last night and wish for contraception

Answers

A1 Emergency contraception is not a substitute for a reliable long-term contraceptive method.

A2 It is important to establish the timing of intercourse, as this will determine the type of post-coital contraception that would be suitable for the patient. Her sexual history, including the number of partners (including casual relationships) should also be sought in order to determine her risk of sexually transmitted diseases (STD).

A3 If there is a risk of STD, then specific examination of the vagina and cervix will be necessary (see case 5.2).

A4 If there is a risk of STD, then specific investigations such as high vaginal and cervical swabs will be needed (see Case 5.2). Otherwise, pelvic examination is not necessary.

A5 EMERGENCY CONTRACEPTION

- The 'morning-after pill' reduces the likelihood of conception at mid-cycle from 15–25% to 1%. It has to be taken within 72 h of the time of last unprotected intercourse. However, hormonal preparations are more effective if they are taken within 24 rather than 72 h.

- The 'Yupze regimen' – two tablets of a combined oral contraceptive pill (equivalent to 100 µg ethinyloestradiol and 500 micrograms levonorgestrel) are taken, and the dose is repeated 12 h later.

- Progesterone-only pills – two tablets of 0.75 mg levonorgestrel (equivalent to 20 tablets of Noegest, 25 tablets of Microval or 25 tablets of Norgesten) are taken 12 h apart and initiated within 72 h of intercourse. This method prevents 89% of expected pregnancies compared to 76% with the combined preparation when taken properly within 72 h.

- If the patient presents after 72 h but within 5 days of intercourse, IUCD insertion will usually prevent implantation.

Table 7.1 *Long-term contraception*

	Advantages	Disadvantages	Mode of action	Failure rates per 100 women years (PEARL index*)	Other comments
Combined oral contraceptive (COC) pill	Good cycle control, reduces menses flow, reduces dysmenorrhoea, and is well accepted. Risks of endometrial and ovarian cancer and endometriosis are reduced. There is also a reduction in morbidity of rheumatoid arthritis, and thyroid disorders	Higher doses have a higher risk of venous thromboembolism, particularly if the woman is a smoker (see below). Also not suitable for those over 40 years, hypertensive and overweight women. Does not protect against STD	Inhibits ovulation by suppressing LH and FSH release	0.16–0.27	Would be suitable for this patient (possibly with condoms as well to reduce her risk from STDs)
Progesterone-only pill (POP)	Safe to use in older women and following pregnancy in lactating women. There are no increased risks of thrombosis	Daily tablet, meticulous timing (± 3 h) is extremely important for it to be effective. Does not protect against STD	Cervical mucus becomes hostile to sperm and can inhibit ovulation in up to 40% of women	2–3	*Depot progestogens have similar mode of action to POP. Injection every 3 months means that compliance is excellent. Can result in troublesome irregular bleeding patterns, but causes prolonged amenorrhoea after long-term use*

Intrauterine contraceptive device (IUCD)	Highly effective and once-only preparation, needing to be changed from every 3 years (Copper) to 5 years (progestogen-impregnated IUCD – Mirena). Latter reduces menstrual blood loss to 97% of cases being amenorrhoeic within 12 months	Both types can result in pelvic infection and perforation	Prevents implantation and therefore considered by some to be an arbortifacient	0.2–0.3	Mirena coil can cause irregular bleeding for up to 6–9 months
Condoms	Protects against all types of sexually transmitted diseases. Essential for casual intercourse	Higher failure rate if not used properly	Barrier method of contraception	3.6	
Cap/diaphragm	Woman has control over contraception, and the method is non-hormonal	Needs well-motivated individual to use it properly. Needs to be inserted before intercourse and removed at least 6 h later. Inconvenient to use and provides limited protection against STDs	Barrier method of contraception	Up to 20	
Natural	Lactation has a major contraceptive role world-wide, as well as having major benefits for the neonate and infant (see OCSE 13.1)	Unreliable, and offers no protection against STDs	'Rhythm' method avoids intercourse during the fertile period around ovulation (i.e. duration depending on maximum sperm (5 days) and ovum (24 h) survival (see OSCE 6.1). 'Withdrawal' involves removal of penis before ejaculation, but sperm can be released before orgasm	Up to 30	

*If the PEARL index is 4, then of 100 women using it for a year, 4 will be pregnant by the end of the year.

Table 7.2 *Disadvantages of the combined oral contraceptive (COC) pill*

	Incidence of thromboembolism per 100 000 women/year using COC
All women not using 'pill'	5
Pregnant women	60
Women using older 30-µg pill	15 (second-generation pill containing levonorgestrel)
Women using new 30-µg pill	25 (third-generation pill containing desogestrel or gestodene)
Women smoking and using pill	60

Case 7.2   My family is complete and I now wish to be sterilized   Answers

A1 The peak age for sterilization requests is between 30 and 34 years. The patient's young age, all male children and recent separation from her husband are factors that could lead her to regret her decision in the future. It is possible that she may have made this decision in reaction to her separation. She might change her mind if she was to be reconciled with her husband, or if she finds a new partner.

A2 Is the patient absolutely certain about her request? The history is targeted to determine the patient's fitness for anaesthesia, to make a choice of operative approach in the light of previous operations, and to explore the cervical smear history. The patient's last menstrual period date should be checked on the day of her admission to ensure that she is not pregnant before surgery.

A3 A cardiovascular and respiratory examination should be performed to assess fitness for anaesthesia. Examination of the abdomen should be made for surgical scars that may increase the risk of intra-abdominal adhesions.

A4
- **FBC** ☑ Fitness for anaesthesia.

- **Urinary pregnancy test** ☑ To exclude pregnancy at the time of admission to hospital before surgery.

- **Cervical smear** ☑ If not done during the last 3 years.

A3 CONSENT AND COUNSELLING

- It must be stressed that the sterilization operation is a permanent and irreversible procedure.

- In general, a 1:200 (0.5%) failure risk is present. In the case of sterilization failure, it is more likely to be an ectopic pregnancy.

- A laparoscopic, day-case procedure with general anaesthetic is used. It involves two small abdominal scars – subumbilical and suprapubic (or iliac fossa). There may be shoulder-tip pain due to abdominal distension with carbon dioxide.

- Although the procedure is very safe, there are inherent risks associated with laparoscopic surgery – primarily visceral damage to the bowel (1.6–1.8 in 1000 cases), bladder and blood vessels (1 in 1000 cases), which may warrant mid-line laparotomy. Consent must therefore be obtained for a laparotomy in the event of complications.

- Check that the patient is certain of her request despite knowing that sterilization will not stabilize an insecure marriage.

- Alternative long-term effective but reversible forms of contraception are available (e.g. IUCD).

- It is possible that the patient will experience heavier periods after stopping the oral contraceptive pill.

- If the couple had still been together, it would be better to obtain consent from both partners and to advise them that the alternative is vasectomy, which is a quicker procedure that is performed under local anaesthetic. However failure rates are higher.

- Agreement to sterilization must never be a prior condition for agreement to undertake termination of pregnancy.

- Childbirth and abortion are both stressful times for the patient, and extra care and time must be given to allow her to reflect the sterilization decision at these times.

The procedure

● Laparoscopic sterilization is a day-case procedure in which any of several different techniques for tubal occlusion are used, including the Filshie clip, Fallope ring and diathermy (unipolar or bipolar). The patient should be advised to use the current form of contraception until the start of the next period after sterilization.

Case 7.3 I am pregnant and don't want to be Answers

A1 A request for termination of an unplanned and unwanted pregnancy (therapeutic abortion) is common. This is usually a result of either poor motivation to use contraceptives or failure of contraception. Reliable contraceptive advice and counselling would therefore be mandatory, as abortion should never be used as a method of contraception.

A2 It would be essential to obtain information about the date of the last normal menstrual period, the menstrual history and cycle regularity in order to establish a gestational age (see Case 9.1). A history of asthma would preclude the use of prostaglandins as a treatment option.

A3 If surgical termination of pregnancy is anticipated, the chest should be examined to assess fitness for anaesthesia. Abdominal examination would also be necessary in order to determine uterine size. A palpable uterus would indicate a gestation of more than 12 weeks.

A4
- **FBC** ☑ To determine the patient's fitness for anaesthesia.
- **Blood group** ☑ To check the patient's rhesus status (if she is rhesus-negative, prophylactic anti-D will be required).
- **USS** ☑ To determine the gestational age accurately.

A4 CONSENT AND COUNSELLING

- It should be made clear that there is a risk of infertility following abortion that could lead to considerable psychological trauma in the future. Psychological morbidity and regret can be considerable, and counselling should be offered as part of the termination service. There is evidence that this psychological morbidity is lower in women who choose medical methods of abortion.

- The complication rates are lower with medical methods, particularly the risk of sepsis (which can lead to future infertility). Perforation of the uterus and visceral damage can occur with surgical methods, but are rare and dependent on the surgeon's expertise.

- The risk of pregnancy is highest in the first 4 weeks following abortion, and therefore adequate contraceptive advice, such as the combined oral contraceptive, Depot gestogens or IUCD, is mandatory. This contraception should preferably be started before the patient is discharged.

- The treatment options are as follows.

MEDICAL

- Up to 9 weeks' gestation, oral mifepristone (an antiprogesterone abortifacient) followed by vaginal prostaglandins administered 36–48 h later would result in complete abortion in 95% of cases. The earlier the gestation, the higher the probability of complete abortion.

- In fact, at gestations of 6 weeks or less, surgical abortion would not be advisable as the pregnancy can be missed. However, before this method is considered, an ultrasound dating of the pregnancy is essential to ensure that the pregnancy is less than 9 completed weeks.

SURGICAL

Surgical evacuation of the uterus, normally with a suction curette, is the commonest method of terminating pregnancy, and is usually performed as a day-case procedure under general anaesthetic. This procedure is safe up to 12 weeks' gestation. In nulliparous women, cervical 'ripening' agents (e.g. prostaglandins, mifepristerone) are essential to soften the cervix prior to cervical dilatation in order to reduce the risk of trauma to the cervix and potential cervical incompetence in the future. The administration of prophylactic antibiotics at the time of termination of pregnancy should be considered.

Box 7.1 Key facts about termination of pregnancy

- Induced abortion is one of the most commonly performed gynaecological procedures in the UK.
- Around 180 000 terminations are performed annually in England and Wales.
- Around 12 000 terminations are performed annually in Scotland.
- At least one-third of women in the UK will have had a termination of pregnancy by the time they reach the age of 45 years.
- Over 98% of terminations in the UK are undertaken because the pregnancy threatens the mental and physical health of the woman or her children.

Case 7.4   I have just had a baby and I now require contraception   Answers

A1 Breastfeeding (lactational amenorrhoea method) is the commonest type of contraception used world-wide. It works by preventing ovulation and causing amenorrhoea. Fully breastfeeding without supplementation provides more than 98% protection until one of three conditions occur – menses return, breastfeeding is reduced, or the baby reaches 6 months of age. This patient requires a more reliable form of contraception than full breastfeeding. The progesterone-only pill is safe to use in lactating women, but is only effective if it is taken religiously. It can cause irregularity of the cycle, which can result in non-compliance. This method failed after the patient's last pregnancy. Thus another reliable form of contraception is necessary to reduce the risk of an unwanted pregnancy. It is possible that ovulation can occur before menses, and therefore it is essential to prescribe a more effective form of contraception almost immediately. The patient's age and the fact that she is breastfeeding are significant factors to consider when choosing an appropriate contraceptive. The combined oral contraceptive is contraindicated in women who are breastfeeding, and it suppresses lactation.

A2 A history of smoking and obesity would increase the patient's risk of venous thromboembolism if she were to be prescribed the combined oral contraceptive. Enquire whether the patient's family is complete, as she might then be a candidate for sterilization.

A3 No specific examination is necessary. Pelvic examination is only required if there are gynaecological symptoms.

A4 No specific investigations are required.

A5 Encourage full breastfeeding, as it has many benefits (see OSCE 13.1). However, the contraceptive benefit of breastfeeding will not be sufficient for this patient. Any of the methods described below will be suitable for her.

- *Depot progestogens (Depo Provera)* – this is a 3-month form of contraception and it is effective if compliance is going to be a problem. It is safe to prescribe for women who are breastfeeding. It can also be used to avoid pregnancy following postnatal rubella vaccination. It can cause irregular bleeding and prolonged amenorrhoea.

- *IUCD* – this is highly effective, particularly in poorly compliant women. It is a long-term but reversible form of contraception, and it is suitable for older women. It can normally be placed after delivery of the placenta or 6 weeks postnatally. There is a very high probability of expulsion in the former case, as the uterus contracts rapidly postnatally. There is also a risk of perforation (due to a soft uterus) and infection in the immediate postpartum period.

- *Sterilization* – when performed at 3 months post-delivery this is known as 'interval laparoscopic sterilization'. If performed immediately postnatally it would require a mini-laparotomy procedure, as the uterus is still enlarged to between 14–16 weeks' size, which does not permit a laparoscopic approach. The latter method needs to be discussed with the parents during early pregnancy to ensure that they are completely happy about the permanent and irreversible nature of the procedure. However, the morbidity to the mother is considerably less at interval sterilization, as it can be performed as a day-case procedure and also allows an adequate safe interval to assess whether the neonate is healthy before proceeding to a permanent form of contraception.

OSCE counselling case 7.1   How should I take 'morning-after' pills?

A 17-year-old university student presents on the morning after having had a condom 'accident'. She is extremely concerned about the possibility of pregnancy, which she feels would be a disaster at this stage in her life. Her last menstrual period was 15 days previously and she has a regular cycle. You decide to prescribe emergency hormonal contraception.

Q1   What instructions would you give her?

OSCE counselling case 7.2   How should I take the pill?

A young single nulliparous girl is requesting the combined oral contraceptive pill. She has never used contraception before, and has no contraindications for use.

Q1   Explain to her how to take the pill, and give her any additional information about missed pills.

OSCE counselling case 7.1   How should I take 'morning-after' pills?

Answers

A1
- There are two forms of emergency hormonal contraception.

  1 The newly licensed progestogen-only emergency contraceptive, Levonelle-2, consists of two tablets of 0.75 mg of levonorgestrel taken 12 h apart. It is more effective and has fewer side-effects (nausea and vomiting in 23% and 6%, respectively) than the combined pill. It is the treatment of choice;

  2 Two tablets of a combined oral contraceptive pill (equivalent to 100 μg of ethinyloestradiol and 500 micrograms of levonorgestrel) are taken, and the dose is repeated 12 h later.

  Nausea and vomiting are common problems (in up to 50% and 20% of cases, respectively) with the combined pill preparation. If the tablets are expelled in the vomitus, treatment may need to be repeated. An anti-emetic could be prescribed simultaneously, and domperidone (10 mg tablet) is the treatment of choice with each dose of hormone.

- Advise the patient to use barrier methods until her next period.

- Warn her that her period may be early or late.

- Advise her that she needs to return for follow-up, whether or not she has a period or light bleed, to ensure that she is not pregnant and that she has effective contraception for the future (choosing one of the options from Table 7.1).

OSCE counselling case 7.2 How should I take the pill?

A1 • Explain how to take the pill.

1 Start on day 1 of the menstrual cycle.

2 Stop after 21 days.

3 Have a 7-day break during which a withdrawal bleed should occur.

4 Restart a new packet for 21 days.

5 Give the patient a leaflet about pill-taking.

• Mention the need for additional protection if the patient has vomiting or diarrhoea or takes antibiotics.

• Indicate what to do if she misses one or more pills.

1 If she misses a pill during the first 14 days, she should take the most recently missed pill and use a condom for 7 days. Then continue as normal.

2 If she misses a pill during the last 7 days, she should take the most recently missed pill, use condoms for 7 days, and start the next packet *without* the usual 7-day break.

3 Give her a leaflet about missed pills.

• Mention the possible minor side-effects (e.g. nausea, lighter 'periods').

• Mention the need for follow-up in 6 months, or earlier if she experiences any problems.

• Advise that the pill does not protect against sexually transmitted diseases.

Part 2

Obstetrics

8 Early pregnancy problems

The clinical cases included in this chapter are as follows:

Case 8.1   My period is 2 weeks late and I am bleeding
Case 8.2   I am 6 weeks pregnant and have pain and bleeding
Case 8.3   I am pregnant and cannot keep anything down

The OSCE counselling cases included in this chapter are as follows:

OSCE counselling case 8.1   I am upset that my first pregnancy has ended up in miscarriage
OSCE counselling case 8.2   This is my third miscarriage. What can be done about it?

In order to work through the core clinical cases in this chapter, you will need to understand the following key concepts.

KEY CONCEPTS

Bleeding in early pregnancy
- Bleeding in early pregnancy is very common (20% of cases).
- 20% of pregnancies undergo miscarriage.
- Awareness of ectopic pregnancy is important in its investigation.

Case 8.1   My period is 2 weeks late and I am bleeding

A 23-year-old nulliparous woman has had 6 weeks of amenorrhoea. She has not been using any contraception. She normally has a regular menstrual cycle every 28 days. A pregnancy home test is positive. She has noticed slight vaginal spotting.

Case 8.2   I am 6 weeks pregnant and have pain and bleeding

A 34-year-old woman presents with a history of 6 weeks of amenorrhoea, abdominal pain and slight vaginal bleeding. She stopped the oral contraceptive pill 2 years ago in order to conceive, and she recently booked an appointment to see her doctor because she was concerned that she was infertile. She has previously had an appendectomy and pelvic inflammatory disease (PID). Recently she has sometimes been feeling dizzy. A home pregnancy test is positive.

Case 8.3   I am pregnant and cannot keep anything down

A 26-year-old primigravida presents at 8 weeks' gestation with a history of nausea and vomiting for the last 2 weeks. However, she now indicates that she is unable to keep any food or drink down.

Questions *for each of the case scenarios given*

Q1 What is the likely differential diagnosis?
Q2 What issues in the given history support the diagnosis?
Q3 What additional features in the history would you seek to support a particular diagnosis?
Q4 What clinical examination would you perform and why?
Q5 What investigations would be most helpful and why?
Q6 What treatment options are appropriate?

Case 8.1 My period is 2 weeks late and I am bleeding   Answers

A1
- Miscarriage (synonym abortion)
  threatened miscarriage;
  inevitable miscarriage;
  incomplete miscarriage;
  complete miscarriage;
  missed abortion.
- Ectopic pregnancy (see Case 8.2).
- Molar pregnancy.

A2 Six weeks of amenorrhoea and a positive pregnancy test, after regular menstrual cycles, indicate an early pregnancy. The small amount of bleeding is a sign that the patient is threatening to have a miscarriage. However, a firm diagnosis can only be established after further investigations.

A3 The degree of bleeding, associated pain and passage of products of conception would indicate the type of miscarriage (see Table 8.1).

Table 8.1 *Summary of key features in the history, examination, investigations and outcome for the different types of miscarriage and ectopic pregnancy*

	History		Examination		Investigation	Management/ outcome
Type of miscarriage	Pain	Bleeding	Cervical os	Uterine size in relation to gestational age	Uterus on ultrasound scan	
Threatened	Slight/none	Slight to moderate	Closed	Consistent	Fetus with heart beat	25% will miscarry
Inevitable	Considerable	Heavy	Open	Small/consistent	Fetus may be alive	Miscarriage is inevitable
Incomplete	Considerable	Heavy. Some fetal tissue parts may have been passed	Open	Small	Some fetal tissue	Will need evacuation of uterus
Complete	Slight at presentation but considerable earlier on	Slight to moderate after heavy loss	Initially open, then closed after miscarriage	Small	Empty	No treatment required
Missed	Absent	Slight	Closed	Consistent or small	Fetus with no heart beat	Will need evacuation of uterus
Molar	Slight/none	Slight to moderate	Closed	Consistent or large	Classical 'snow-storm' appearance of vesicles	Will need evacuation of uterus and follow-up
Ectopic	None/slight	Slight	Closed/tender	Small	Empty uterus	See Case 8.2

A4 Assess the patient's haemodynamic status, including blood pressure, pulse and degree of bleeding. An abdominal examination is essential to elicit signs of rebound tenderness and acute abdomen (ectopic pregnancy).

Speculum examination should be performed to visualize the cervical os and determine whether fetal tissue is present in the os or in the vagina. The nature of the cervical os (open/closed) on digital examination will help to distinguish between the different types of miscarriage. Uterine size should be assessed during bimanual examination. Uterine tenderness is unlikely unless there is septic abortion. Vaginal examination may elicit cervical excitation and adnexal tenderness in ectopic pregnancy.

A5

- **Urine βHCG** ✓ To confirm pregnancy. Home pregnancy tests may be unreliable.

- **FBC** ✓ To assess blood loss.

- **Blood group** ± To check rhesus status (if the patient is rhesus-negative, prophylactic anti-D is given).

- **Group and save, cross-match** ✓ In cases of shock.

- **USS** ✓ To determine whether the fetus is intrauterine and if it is viable. It will also detect retained fetal tissue (products of conception). The absence of intrauterine fetal tissue (i.e. empty uterus) should suggest the possibility of an ectopic pregnancy.

- **Serum βHCG** ✓ There is a doubling of levels within 48 h in a viable intrauterine pregnancy.

- **Histology** ✓ Any tissue expelled from the uterus should be sent for histology to exclude molar pregnancy. Sometimes the tissue is an endometrial cast without any trophoblast, indicating an ectopic pregnancy.

A6 **CONSERVATIVE**

Bed-rest does not prevent miscarriage. Admission to hospital in cases of threatened abortion is not always necessary.

MEDICAL

Intramuscular ergometrine may be required to reduce heavy bleeding in cases of incomplete, inevitable or complete abortion. In patients with mild bleeding it may be possible to avoid surgical evacuation in incomplete miscarriage by using mifepristone and prostaglandins to induce evacuation of the uterus. This treatment is currently still being evaluated for its efficacy.

SURGICAL

Removal of fetal tissue from the os can stop uncontrollable bleeding. In incomplete or missed abortion, evacuation of retained products of conception under general anaesthetic is used to prevent continued bleeding and the risk of infection.

Case 8.2 I am 6 weeks pregnant and have pain and bleeding Answers

A1
- Ectopic pregnancy.
- Miscarriage (see Case 8.1).

A2 Diagnosing ectopic pregnancy can be difficult. A period of amenorrhoea, abdominal/pelvic pain and slight bleeding is classically associated with ectopic pregnancy. Syncopal episodes (fainting /dizziness) are associated with Fallopian tube distension and stimulation of the autonomic nervous system. Previous surgery (e.g. appendectomy), pelvic inflammatory disease and conception after infertility are all risk factors for ectopic pregnancy.

A3 Any factors which may damage the Fallopian tubes are risk factors for ectopic pregnancy, including PID secondary to sexually transmitted disease or IUCD (but also by the mechanism whereby IUCDs prevent intrauterine implantation). Tubal surgery such as reversal of sterilization (8% risk of ectopic pregnancy) and salpingostomy for hydrosalpinges, and assisted conception (e.g. IVF) are additional risk factors. Other symptoms include shoulder-tip pain due to irritation of the diaphragm by blood leaking from the ectopic.

A4 Assessment of the patient's haemodynamic stability by checking blood pressure (to detect hypotension) and pulse (to detect tachycardia) will indicate the degree of blood loss. An abdominal examination should be performed to elicit tenderness to palpation, rebound tenderness, guarding or rigidity, as well as gentle vaginal examination to detect cervical excitation (pelvic tenderness on moving the cervix) and the possibility of palpating a tender adnexal mass. Care should be taken not to convert an unruptured stable ectopic to an emergency situation by compressing and rupturing an ectopic mass bimanually during vaginal examination.

A5
- **Urine βHCG** ✓ This should always be tested in women of reproductive age who present with pain and bleeding, to confirm pregnancy.

- **FBC** ✓ To assess the systemic effect of bleeding.

- **Blood group** ✓ To check the patient's rhesus status (if rhesus-negative, prophylactic anti-D is given).

- **Group and save, cross-match** ✓ In cases of shock.

- **Serum βHCG** ✓ Normally a doubling of levels in 48 h is associated with intrauterine pregnancy. This test should be undertaken if conservative management is planned in a stable patient.

- **USS (preferably transvaginal)** ✓ This can indicate an intrauterine pregnancy as early as 6 weeks' amenorrhoea. An empty uterus, fluid in the pouch of Douglas and an adnexal mass on ultrasound scan would give a high index of suspicion of ectopic pregnancy.

- **Diagnostic laparoscopy** ✓ This is the gold standard for confirming the diagnosis. Very early ectopics can still be missed at laparoscopy. The false-negative rate is about 5%.

A6 CONSERVATIVE

There is no place for conservative management in ectopic pregnancy if the patient is *symptomatic*, as this is a life-threatening condition. The patient should be admitted to hospital and definitive treatment administered.

A conservative approach would only be appropriate if the patient was asymptomatic and, after investigations, there was uncertainty about the diagnosis. A very early intrauterine pregnancy may not be visible on a scan, but βHCG repeated after 48 h would show a doubling of levels if the pregnancy was viable. If the pregnancy is not viable, βHCG levels will fall and will eventually become non-detectable.

MEDICAL

Unruptured ectopics less than 3–4 cm in size can be treated with methotrexate systematically (or by administering it into the ectopic sac under USS or laparoscopic guidance). Follow-up with βHCG is essential, as the risk of persistent ectopic pregnancy is high. This method may allow the tube to function, as 60% of women will subsequently have a successful pregnancy. There is a 15% risk of recurrent ectopic pregnancy.

SURGICAL

This may involve laparoscopy or laparotomy.

- Milking of the ectopic or salpingotomy can be used for removal of an ectopic pregnancy without removing the tube. Both of these procedures salvage the tube, but follow-up with βHCGs is essential to look for persistent ectopic pregnancy.

- Salpingectomy involves removal of the ectopic with the tube. Follow-up with βHCG is not necessary in this case.

Case 8.3 I am pregnant and cannot keep anything down Answers

A1
- Hyperemesis gravidarum (multiple pregnancy, molar pregnancy, thyrotoxicosis).
- Urinary tract infection (UTI).
- Appendicitis.
- Gastrointestinal infection.
- Rarer problems (e.g. bowel obstruction, hepatic disorders or cerebral tumours).

A2 Pregnancy and vomiting of all food and drink support the diagnosis of hyperemesis, particularly in the first trimester.

A3 Acute onset of the problem would support a diagnosis such as gastroenteritis or appendicitis. A longer duration of the symptoms with pre-existing nausea/vomiting would support a diagnosis of hyperemesis. Associated symptoms (e.g. diarrhoea, urinary symptoms, abdominal pain), other members of the family with the same problem, and symptoms of thyrotoxicosis would support a diagnosis other than hyperemesis.

A4 Look for evidence of dehydration (e.g. dry mouth, tachycardia or postural hypotension). Abdominal signs of tenderness and guarding would support a diagnosis of appendicitis. A large-for-dates uterus would suggest multiple pregnancy as a cause of hyperemesis.

A5
- **FBC** [✓] Haemoglobin for haemoconcentration and white cell count (WCC) for infection.
- **U&E** [✓] To check for dehydration.
- **MSU** [✓] To exclude urinary tract infection.
- **Urinalysis** [✓] The presence of ketones supports a history of excessive vomiting.
- **USS** [✓] To exclude molar and multiple pregnancy.
- **LFT** [±] For liver disorders.
- **TSH** [±] To exclude thyrotoxicosis. Note that TSH can be suppressed in hyperemesis.

A6 Conditions other than hyperemesis require treatment specific to the problem (e.g. evacuate molar pregnancy with appropriate follow-up (urinary and serum βHCGs and avoiding pregnancy with adequate contraception until normal βHCGs have been obtained); appendectomy for appendicitis).

Hyperemesis

SUPPORTIVE

- Admit the patient to hospital.

- Reassure her that this problem is likely to resolve spontaneously at 12–14 weeks when βHCG levels start to decline.

- Offer psychological support (many women have additional social and emotional problems).

MEDICAL

- Intravenous fluids.

- Anti-emetics (prochlorperazine, IM, suppository; metoclopramide, IM; ondansetron, IV).

- Introduce foods as appropriate in small amounts – avoid fatty foods.

- Steroids may be given in severe cases.

- Vitamin supplementation (vitamin B6 if prolonged vomiting occurs).

- May occasionally require parenteral nutrition.

SURGICAL

- In severe cases, termination of pregnancy may need to be considered.

I am upset that my first pregnancy has ended up in a miscarriage

A 23-year-old woman has had an evacuation of the uterus following an incomplete abortion at 10 weeks' gestation in her first pregnancy. She is ready for discharge home and is very upset.

Q1 What counselling would you give her about miscarriage and about post-operative recovery prior to discharge?

OSCE counselling case 8.2 This is my third miscarriage. What can be done about it?

A patient has just undergone an evacuation of the uterus for her third consecutive spontaneous abortion. She has had no pregnancies beyond 10 weeks' gestation.

Q1 What investigations should be undertaken?

Q2 In the absence of any identifiable cause, what are her chances of achieving an ongoing pregnancy on the next occasion?

A1 *Miscarriage*
- Miscarriage is very common, with approximately 1 in 5 pregnancies ending in miscarriage.
- Most are unexplained.
- There is nothing that the patient could have done that would have caused the miscarriage.
- There is nothing that she could have done to prevent the miscarriage.
- Her risk of miscarriage in the next pregnancy is not increased.

Post-operative recovery
- The patient can expect some continued vaginal blood loss for a few days. It should not be heavy or offensive, and should gradually tail off. If the loss becomes heavy and fresh or offensive, she should seek medical help.
- There is no medical reason why she needs to delay further attempts at pregnancy, but she must feel psychologically ready. You might suggest waiting for one normal period.
- If she needs additional support, offer her contact telephone numbers and information about early pregnancy loss support groups within the local area. In addition, you might offer a follow-up appointment if she would find this helpful.
- If she is rhesus-negative, ensure that she has had anti-D prior to discharge, and explain the reasons for this.

OSCE counselling case 8.2 This is my third miscarriage. What can be done about it?

Answers

A1
- Three consecutive abortions are defined as recurrent abortion. The latter is more often associated with an identifiable cause than are isolated cases of miscarriage.
- Investigations would include the following:

  1 chromosomal analysis of the products of conception;

  2 chromosomal analysis of both parents – a chromosomal abnormality (e.g. balanced translocation) will be diagnosed in one of the partners in 5–7% of cases of recurrent abortion;

  3 maternal blood for anticardiolipin antibodies and lupus anticoagulant.

A2 There is a 60–70% likelihood of successful pregnancy if no cause is found for recurrent abortions.

The clinical cases included in this chapter are as follows:
Case 9.1 I think that I am pregnant, but I cannot remember the date of my last menstrual period
Case 9.2 The midwife says my baby is small
Case 9.3 The midwife says my baby is big

The OSCE counselling cases included in this chapter are as follows:
OSCE counselling case 9.1 I have been told that my baby is small. How am I going to be monitored?
OSCE counselling case 9.2 I want to have screening for Down's Syndrome. What is involved?

In order to work through the core clinical cases in this chapter, you will need to understand the following key concepts.

KEY CONCEPTS

Small for gestational age (SGA) (see Figure 9.1)
Term used to describe a fetus with a birth weight of < 10th centile for gestation. This may reflect:
a fetus that is growing normally but constitutionally small; or
chronic compromise due to 'placental insufficiency' leading to intrauterine growth restriction.

Intrauterine growth restriction (IUGR) (see Figure 9.2)
Term used to describe a fetus that has failed to achieve its growth potential (i.e. if a fetus is genetically determined to be 3.8 kg but only achieves 2.8 kg).

Viability
Taken to be after 24 completed weeks in the UK.

Large for dates
Term used to describe a fetus with a birth weight of > 95th centile for gestational age.

Polyhydramnios
Excess amniotic fluid (> 8 cm average liquor pocket depth on ultrasound, but is dependent on gestational age).

Macrosomia
Birth weight of > 4.5 kg.

Oligohydramnios
Reduced amniotic fluid (< 2 cm average liquor pocket depth on ultrasound).

Term
Pregnancy between 37 and 42 completed gestational weeks.

Preterm
Pregnancy before 37 completed gestational weeks.

Post-term
Pregnancy beyond 42 completed gestational weeks.

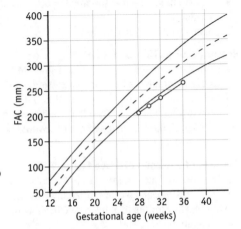

Figure 9.1 *Fetal abdominal circumference (FAC) in an SGA fetus with normal growth (constitutionally small).*

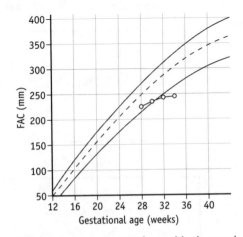

Figure 9.2 *FAC in an SGA fetus with abnormal growth (IUGR).*

Gravida

Number of pregnancies, including current pregnancy.

Parity

Two figures are given. The first is the number of pregnancies beyond 24 weeks plus those ending before 24 weeks in which there were signs of life, and the second is the number of pregnancies ending before 24 weeks without signs of life.

Box 9.1 *Cardiotocography (CTG)*

Components of a CTG

A cardiotocograph is a combined pictorial representation of the continuous recording made up of two components:

- '*Cardio*' component – fetal heart trace measured by external ultrasound sonicaid, or best obtained by an electrode attached to the fetal scalp (or fetal buttock);
- '*Toco*' component – measurement of uterine contraction activity assessed by external strain gauge transducer.

The paper speed is set at 1 cm/min.

Reasons why a CTG is performed

- During the antenatal period, a 'non-stress test' (when no contractions are expected) by a cardiotocograph is a method of assessing fetal well-being.
- During the intrapartum period, continuous recording is used to detect 'fetal distress', with the aim of detecting fetal hypoxia. The effects of hypoxia depend on fetal glycogen reserves. A growth-retarded fetus which has less glycogen reserves would be affected earlier and more severely than a well-nourished fetus.

Features of a normal CTG (see Figure 9.3)

- The baseline rate can range from 110 to 150 beats/min (bpm) for a term fetus.
- The 'beat-to-beat' baseline variability is 10–25 beats/min. This indicates a 'reactive' trace. It is normal and healthy for the fetal heart rate to show this degree of irregularity.
- There are no decelerations.
- There are at least two accelerations (> 15 beats/min for 15 s) in a 20-min trace.
- There is an indication of when fetal movements have occurred, which the mother has electronically added to the trace.

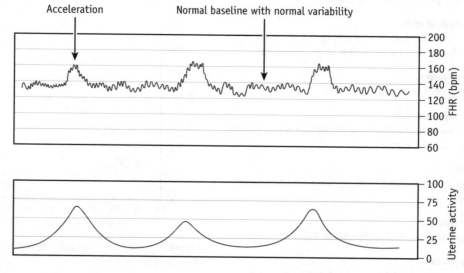

Figure 9.3 *Features of a normal CTG.*

Types of abnormalities that a CTG can detect

- *Early deceleration* – deceleration beginning with the onset of the contraction, returning to the baseline rate by the end of the contraction, and usually < 40 beats/min. Can be due to head compression, cord compression or early hypoxia (see Figure 9.4).
- *Variable deceleration* – deceleration appearing at a variable time during the contraction, of irregular shape and > 50 beats/min often caused by cord compression.
- *Late deceleration* – deceleration trough is the lowest point, which is past the peak of the contraction (the lag time). Late decelerations are associated with fetal hypoxia. The worst scenario is a combination of several features (i.e. loss of beat-to-beat variability, tachycardia of > 160 beats/min and late decelerations) This appearance is strongly associated with fetal hypoxia (see Figure 9.5).

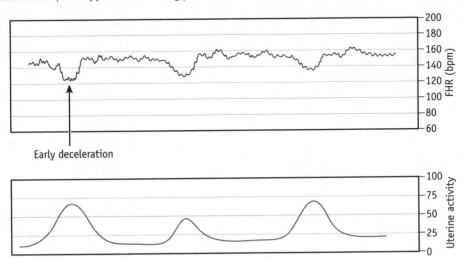

Figure 9.4 *Abnormal CTG – early decelerations.*

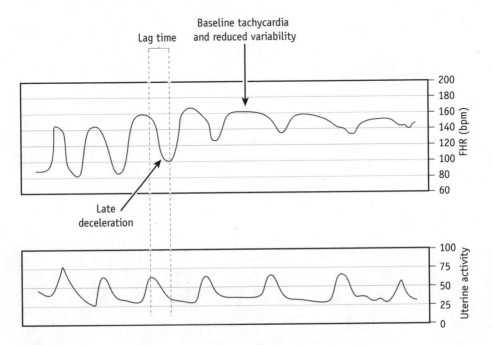

Figure 9.5 *Abnormal CTG – late decelerations/tachycardia/reduced variability.*

Case 9.1   I think I am pregnant, but I cannot remember the date of my last menstrual period

A 23-year-old woman has a positive pregnancy test but is uncertain about the exact stage of her pregnancy. She thinks that her last period was 4 months ago. She has had irregular and infrequent periods in the past. She has presented for her first antenatal visit, and this is her first pregnancy.

Case 9.2   The midwife says my baby is small

A 28-year-old schoolteacher in her second pregnancy attends the midwife antenatal clinic at 32 weeks' gestation. There are adequate fetal movements, but the midwife is concerned that the uterus feels small for dates. The symphysio–fundal height is 27 cm. The patient is a smoker and admits to smoking 20 cigarettes per day. Her antenatal care to date has been uneventful.

Case 9.3   The midwife says my baby is big

A 32-year-old woman in her third pregnancy attends the midwife antenatal clinic at 34 weeks' gestation. The midwife is concerned that the uterus feels large for dates. A booking scan had shown a singleton pregnancy consistent with menstrual dates. The symphysio–fundal height measures 40 cm. There were no anomalies noted on her 20-week scan. The patient has experienced increasing abdominal discomfort during the last 2 weeks, and she is having irregular uterine activity. In addition, she has noticed an increase in shortness of breath.

Questions *for each of the case scenarios given*

Q1   What is the likely differential diagnosis?
Q2   What issues in the given history support the diagnosis?
Q3   What additional features in the history would you seek to support a particular diagnosis?
Q4   What clinical examination would you perform and why?
Q5   What investigations would be most helpful and why?
Q6   What treatment options are appropriate?

Case 9.1 I think I am pregnant, but I cannot remember the date of my last menstrual period

A1 Uncertain dates – pregnancy dating is crucial in this patient's further management, as prenatal biochemical screening for Down's syndrome is dependent on gestational age. Furthermore, decisions about the type and frequency of antenatal care, as well as decisions about delivery, particularly post-term delivery, are also dependent on pregnancy dating.

A2 The irregular infrequent periods support the dating uncertainty. The first day of the last menstrual period (LMP) is usually used to calculate the estimated date of delivery (EDD) (e.g. by the obstetric 'wheel'). This is reserved for a 28-day cycle, assuming that ovulation occurs 14 days after the last menstrual period. A longer cycle would require an upward adjustment of the EDD by the number of days that the cycle is longer than 28 days (e.g. adding 7 days if the cycle length is 35 days).

A3 A detailed menstrual history should be obtained, as well as a history of contraceptive use (e.g. recent use of the combined pill or Depo-Provera, which may make ovulation timing unpredictable after cessation of contraception).

A4
- General health and nutritional status (gestational diabetes is more common in overweight women).
- Height (dystocia is more common in short (< 150 cm) women).
- Baseline blood pressure.
- Chest examination (to identify previously undiagnosed heart murmers).
- Breast examination (to detect incidental breast disease).
- The patient's abdomen should be palpated in order to determine the pregnancy size. The uterus is usually palpable abdominally at 12–14 weeks' gestation. The fundus reaches the umbilicus at 20 weeks' gestation. Thereafter, each additional gestational week is measured as a 1-cm increase in the symphysio–fundal height (see Figure 9.6).

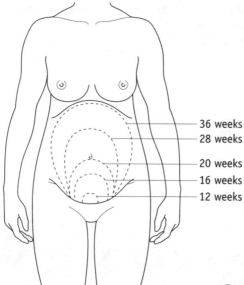

36 weeks
28 weeks
20 weeks
16 weeks
12 weeks

Figure 9.6 *Uterine size in pregnancy.*

A5
- **Urinalysis** ✓

- **Urine culture** ✓ (Asymptomatic bacteriuria can lead to pyelonephritis).

- **FBC** ✓

- **Rhesus and antibody screen** ✓

- **Timed plasma glucose** ✓

- **Serology for syphilis** ✓

- **Rubella IgG** ✓

- **USS** ✓ An ultrasound scan is mandatory in this case, and would be the most accurate way of dating this pregnancy. The fetal crown–rump length is an accurate measurement up to 12 weeks' gestation. The biparietal diameter (BPD) is used between 14–20 weeks. After 20 weeks, growth patterns differ between fetuses, and there is no accurate measurement that reflects gestational age. Other advantages of ultrasound are exclusion of multiple pregnancies, maternal reassurance and detection of fetal structural abnormalities.

- Consider:
  Down's syndrome screening;
  HIV screening;
  hepatitis B;
  haemoglobin electrophoresis for at-risk individuals (e.g. those from Mediterranean region and Asia).

A6 Subsequent antenatal care should be provided as for a normal pregnancy.

Case 9.2   The midwife says my baby is small

A1
- Small for gestational age (SGA) – normally growing but constitutionally small fetus.
- Intrauterine growth restriction (IUGR).
- Wrong dates.

A2
The uterus measurement being small for dates supports SGA or IUGR. Heavy smoking is known to be associated with IUGR.

A2
Checking the certainty of the patient's dates is essential (i.e. accuracy of menstrual data, and findings on ultrasound scans in first and second trimester). This is because if the pregnancy is not as advanced as was believed, this could explain the discrepancy between the symphysio–fundal height and gestational age. Additional risk factors for IUGR are a previous small-for-dates baby, maternal illness (e.g. hypertension), maternal infection in pregnancy (e.g. rubella, cytomegalovirus), increased risk of Down's syndrome screening and history of antepartum haemorrhage.

A2
Examination would include blood pressure measurement to exclude hypertension and pre-eclampsia, which are both associated with IUGR. A clinical assessment of liquor volume should be made because IUGR can be associated with reduced liquor volume. The fetal heart should be auscultated because fetal compromise is associated with IUGR.

A5
- **Urinalysis** ☑ Proteinuria indicates pre-eclampsia if blood pressure is high.

- **Cardiotoc-** ☑ To identify evidence of fetal compromise.
  graphy

- **Ultrasound** ☑ This should be performed (1) to measure abdominal circumference and
  scan   biparietal diameter in order to confirm SGA, (2) to assess liquor volume, (3) to perform umbilical arterial Doppler assessment and (4) to perform a biophysical profile. Ultrasound may also indicate features of congenital infection (brain calcification) or structural anomaly (cardiac defect).

- **Amino-** ☐±☐ This may be considered if there are features on the ultrasound scan that
  centesis or   support a chromosomal anomaly.
  chorionic villus
  sample

- **Fetal blood** ☐±☐ This is only performed in fetal medicine centres. It may be useful if congenital
  sample   infection is suspected.
  (cordocentesis)

A6
The mainstay of management is to deliver as mature a fetus as possible in as good a condition as possible.

- Serial ultrasound examination should be performed to monitor the velocity of fetal growth in order to distinguish between a constitutionally small fetus and an IUGR fetus. The fetus that is growing and not showing evidence of compromise does not require any intervention.

- Umbilical Doppler waveform patterns and biophysical assessment, including cardiotocography, are required to identify evidence of fetal compromise.

- Specific aetiological conditions need appropriate management (e.g. hypertension).

- Steroids to promote surfactant production and reduce the risk or severity of respiratory distress syndrome in the case of preterm delivery.

Box 9.2 *Risks of IUGR and SGA*

Antepartum
- Hypoxia
- Intrauterine death

Peripartum
- Hypoxia
- Intrauterine death
- Meconium aspiration

Postpartum
- Neonatal hypoglycaemia
- Hypocalcaemia
- Hypothermia
- Polycythaemia
- Hypoxic–ischaemic encephalopathy
- Developmental delay and cerebral palsy

Case 9.3   The midwife says my baby is big

A1
- Constitutionally large for dates (LFD).
- Polyhydramnios.
- Wrong dates.
- Multiple pregnancy.
- Macrosomia (e.g. secondary to diabetes).
- Hydrops.

A2
The uterus is clinically large for dates based on symphysio–fundal height. The increased discomfort, irritable uterus and shortness of breath suggest polyhydramnios. The previous dating and second-trimester ultrasound scans have excluded multiple pregnancy and fetal anomaly which might be associated with polyhydramnios (e.g. duodenal atresia).

A3
A family history (e.g. first-degree relative with insulin-dependent diabetes) or maternal obesity increase the risk of gestational diabetes and macrosomia.

Previous high birth weights would support a fetus that is constitutionally large for dates. Rhesus factor and antibody checks are needed to exclude rhesus isoimmunization, which may be associated with fetal hydrops.

A4
Abdominal palpation is necessary to assess liquor volume. A tense uterus, difficulty in feeling fetal parts and fluid thrill all support an increased liquor volume.

A5
- **Glucose tolerance test (GTT)**   ☑   Fasting level > 5.5 mmol/L and 2-h level > 9.0 mmol/L would support a diagnosis of gestational diabetes.

- **USS**   ☑   To:
  1 confirm large for dates [BPD, abdominal circumference];
  2 measure liquor volume;
  3 exclude multiple pregnancy;
  4 exclude fetal anomaly which may have been missed on earlier scans. The fetal micturition and swallowing mechanism is essential to maintain normal liquor volume. Gut atresia is associated with polyhydramnios, as liquor cannot be swallowed;
  5 identify evidence of hydrops (e.g. fetal oedema/effusions and/or ascites).

- **Rhesus status and antibodies**   ☑   To exclude rhesus isoimmunization.

A6
- If gestational diabetes is diagnosed, it should be managed with dietary control and insulin if appropriate.

- Polyhydramnios without symptoms and without evidence of fetal anomaly does not require any treatment. In cases near term where there is maternal discomfort, induction of labour should be considered.

- In cases where the fetus is premature and maternal discomfort is a problem, serial amniocentesis may be considered. However, there is a risk of preterm labour and infection, and the fluid rapidly re-accumulates.

- Indomethacin can reduce liquor volume, but the risk to the fetus is premature closure of the ductus arteriosus and reduced cerebral perfusion.

- If preterm delivery is anticipated, steroids should be given to the mother to promote lung maturity and reduce the risk of respiratory distress syndrome.

Box 9.3 *Risks of polyhydramnios*

- Preterm labour
- Preterm rupture of membranes
- Cord prolapse
- Unstable lie
- Malpresentation
- Abruptio placenta
- Postpartum haemorrhage

OSCE counselling case 9.1   I have been told that my baby is small. How am I going to be monitored?

A woman in her first pregnancy attends the antenatal clinic at 32 weeks. On examination the uterus feels small for dates, and an ultrasound scan confirms that the abdominal circumference is below the fifth centile for gestation. The liquor volume is reported to be within normal limits, and the umbilical Doppler is normal. The woman reports that the baby is active.

Q1 Counsel this patient about the findings and how you propose to monitor fetal well-being.

OSCE counselling case 9.2   I want to have screening for Down's syndrome. What is involved?

A 24-year-old primigravida at 10 weeks' gestation attends the antenatal clinic. She has read about a blood test for Down's syndrome in a magazine, and wishes to discuss this with you.

Q1 Counsel her about biochemical screening for Down's syndrome.

OSCE counselling case 9.1   I have been told that my baby is small. How am I going to be monitored?   **Answers**

A1 Counselling would involve the following points:

- The scan suggests that the baby is small.

- The scan is otherwise normal (normal blood flow measurements and amount of fluid around the baby), and the baby is active.

- It could therefore be that the baby is small and healthy, but it is important to monitor the baby in case the placenta is not working as well as it should and the baby becomes distressed.

- This monitoring will include assessment of the baby's heart beat by external cardiotocography (i.e. a belt attached around her abdomen, which will monitor the heart over a 20-min period). This will be performed every day, but could be done as an out-patient.

- A repeat ultrasound scan will be performed in 1 week to measure blood flow through the umbilical cord (umbilical arterial Doppler), and in 2 weeks to measure how much the baby has grown and again to measure blood flow through the umbilical cord and the amount of fluid around the baby. It is important that the latter is done to check the growth velocity.

- The mother should monitor the movements of the baby and notify the hospital if there is any change in pattern, particularly a reduction in movements.

- If any concern arises about the condition of the baby whilst this monitoring is being undertaken (e.g. signs of fetal distress or inadequate growth), early delivery may be required.

- The mother will be given a course of steroids to help to mature the baby's lungs in case early delivery is indicated.

OSCE counselling case 9.2 I want to have screening for Down's syndrome. What is involved?   **Answers**

A1 Details of the test should include the following:

- what is involved (a venous blood sample);

- when it is performed (15–20 weeks);

- the fact that an ultrasound scan needs to be performed to confirm dates (serum levels of αFP and βHCG are related to gestational age);

- how long the results will take to be returned;

- how the patient will receive the results.

- The test measures αFP and βHCG (αFP is typically low and βHCG is high compared to the population median value in affected pregnancies), and combined with the mother's age will give a measure of her personal risk of having a Down's syndrome baby. The risk is classified as high (> 1:250) or low (< 1:250).

- The test does not diagnose Down's syndrome, and if the patient is in the high-risk category, she will require further investigation (i.e. amniocentesis or chorionic villus sampling – CVS). Both of these tests are associated with excess fetal loss (1% for amniocentesis and 2–3% for CVS).

- If the patient is in the low-risk category, she may still have a baby with Down's syndrome.

- Measurement of nuchal thickness by ultrasound examination in the first trimester, combined with biochemical screening, is another option for screening.

- A detailed anomaly scan at 18–20 weeks may identify associated anomalies (e.g. cardiac abnormalities or other 'markers' for Down's syndrome).

- If the patient had a Down's syndrome fetus, would she consider termination of pregnancy? This may affect her decision as to whether or not to participate in the screening programme.

10 Late pregnancy problems

The clinical cases included in this chapter are as follows:
   Case 10.1   I am 38 weeks pregnant and bleeding vaginally
   Case 10.2   I have not felt my baby move since yesterday
   Case 10.3   I am 32 weeks pregnant and am having contractions

The OSCE counselling cases included in this chapter are as follows:
   OSCE counselling case 10.1   I have experienced bleeding in pregnancy. How will I be managed?
   OSCE counselling case 10.2   How should I record fetal movements?

Case 10.1   I am 38 weeks pregnant and bleeding vaginally

A 24-year-old woman attends the midwife at 38 weeks' gestation. She has had two previous uncomplicated deliveries, and she is concerned that over the past few days she has been having a small amount of fresh vaginal bleeding intermittently. She has no abdominal pain and the baby is active.

Case 10.2   I have not felt my baby move since yesterday

A 30-year-old parous woman at 36 weeks' gestation has not felt any fetal movements on the day when she presents to the doctor. Fetal movements had been becoming less frequent over the last few days, but she had not been recording them. She previously had two normal deliveries at term of babies of normal weight. In this pregnancy her scans showed a singleton fetus consistent with menstrual dates at 12 weeks and with no fetal anomaly at 20 weeks. Her screening for Down's syndrome showed low risk. She has been managed as a low-risk patient, as her pregnancy has progressed without any problems.

Case 10.3   I am 32 weeks pregnant and am having contractions

A 25-year-old nulliparous woman at 32 weeks' gestation presents with abdominal pain associated with uterine contractions. Fetal movements are satisfactory. Her booking ultrasound scan showed singleton pregnancy consistent with menstrual dates and her anomaly scan at 20 weeks' gestation was normal. Her screening for Down's syndrome showed low risk. She had been a smoker but stopped in mid-trimester. She had an appendectomy as a child. She was assessed to be a low-risk pregnancy at booking.

Questions *for each of the case scenarios given*

Q1   What is the likely differential diagnosis?
Q2   What issues in the given history support the diagnosis?
Q3   What additional features in the history would you seek to support a particular diagnosis?
Q4   What clinical examination would you perform and why?
Q5   What investigations would be most helpful and why?
Q6   What treatment options are appropriate?

A1
- Placenta praevia (see Figure 10.1).
- Placental abruption.
- Cervical lesion (e.g. erosion, polyp, cancer).

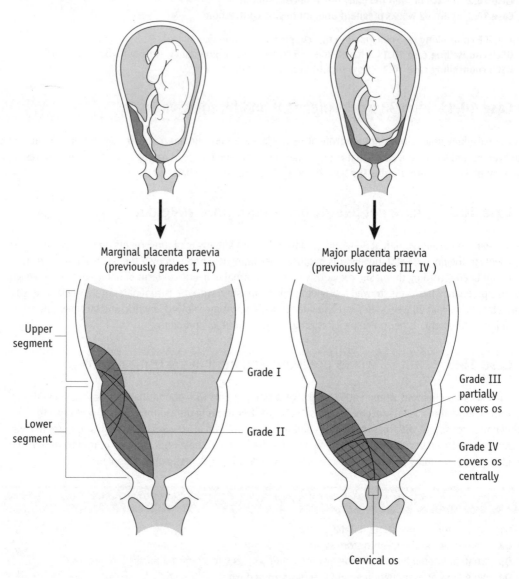

Figure 10.1 *Grades of placenta praevia.*

A2   The history of painless small bleeds supports the diagnosis of placenta praevia.

A3   The patient's smear history should be obtained. The reports of any previous ultrasound scans in this pregnancy should be checked in order to identify the location of the placenta.

A4 The pulse and blood pressure should be recorded.
- Examination would include abdominal palpation, with a soft non-tender uterus, high presenting part and an abnormal lie supporting a diagnosis of placenta praevia, and a tense tender uterus supporting a diagnosis of placental abruption.
- The fetal heart should be auscultated to exclude fetal distress, which is more commonly associated with placental abruption.
- If it is confirmed that the placenta is not low (by ultrasound scan), a speculum examination to visualize the cervix would be indicated. *Under no circumstances should a digital examination be performed*, because torrential bleeding can be provoked if a placenta praevia has falsely been excluded as a cause.

A5
- **FBC** ☑ To identify the presence of anaemia.

- **Blood group and cross-match** ☑ In case bleeding increases and a transfusion is required. The patient should be given anti-D if her blood group is rhesus-negative to prevent isoimmunization.

- **USS** ☑ To localize the placenta and determine whether it is low-lying, as well as to assess fetal growth and well-being.

- **CTG** ☑ To identify suspected fetal compromise.

A6 Management would be to admit the patient to an obstetric unit. At term gestation with a history of antepartum haemorrhage, delivery is indicated to ensure the safe delivery of a mature fetus.

- Caesarean section should be performed in cases of major placenta praevia.

- Consider examination without anaesthesia and artificial rupture of membranes in cases with minor degrees of placenta praevia. This procedure should be performed in an operating-theatre with a senior anaesthetist present and ready to administer a general anaesthetic to expedite delivery if bleeding is provoked on vaginal examination. In addition, cross-matched blood should be available in the operating-theatre and scrub nurses should be ready to perform an immediate Caesarean section (i.e. scrubbed with instrument tray open).

- If a diagnosis of placental abruption is suspected and there is no evidence of fetal compromise, an artificial rupture of the membranes should be performed and a syntocinon infusion commenced with continuous monitoring of the fetal heart.

Box 10.1 *Risks of antepartum haemorrhage*

- Haemorrhage and shock
- Renal failure
- Disseminated intravascular coagulation (DIC)
- Fetal hypoxia
- Intrauterine death

Case 10.2 I have not felt my baby move since yesterday

A1
- Prolonged periods of fetal sleep without any compromise.
- Fetal compromise.
- Fetal death.

A2
In most cases with the given history there is no particular obstetric problem. In this case, the pregnancy had been uncomplicated. Reduced movements had been reported over several days, which would warrant further investigation in order to exclude fetal compromise or death.

A3
The history should explore whether there are any reasons (e.g. hypertension, diabetes, fetal growth retardation and haemorrhage) for concern about fetal compromise.

A4
A general examination, including pulse, temperature (sepsis associated with intrauterine fetal death) and blood pressure (associated pre-eclampsia), is required. The abdomen should be examined to determine the symphysio–fundal height, and clinical assessment of liquor volume should be made (fetal compromise is associated with growth restriction and reduced liquor volume). Try to stimulate fetal movements by gently moving the fetus around at the time of abdominal palpation. Listen to the fetal heart to exclude fetal death (if you hear silence this will need to be confirmed by ultrasound).

A5
- **CTG**   ✓   Cardiotocography to assess fetal well-being, looking for variability, accelerations and a lack of decelerations.

- **USS**   ±   Ultrasound is only required if there is concern about fetal growth or well-being, to (1) check fetal heart rate and (2) assess fetal well-being by assessing liquor volume, fetal movements (which may not be perceived by the patient), fetal tone, fetal respiration and umbilical Doppler (absent or reversed diastolic flow).

A6
- Confirm fetal well-being, and if this is satisfactory then the patient can be discharged home with advice to record fetal movements daily (using a kick chart). If there are less than 10 movements over a 12-h period, the patient will need to return for cardiotocography.

- If there is fetal growth retardation, then investigations will have to be performed to determine the cause. In addition, as the pregnancy is approaching term, delivery may be contemplated.

- If there is fetal death, then medical termination of pregnancy should be conducted together with appropriate investigation (fetal post-mortem, chromosome analysis of fetus and parents, anticardiolipin antibodies and infection screen) and bereavement counselling.

Case 10.3   I am 32 weeks pregnant and am having contractions   Answers

A1
- Obstetric causes:
  - preterm labour;
  - chorionamnionitis;
  - concealed abruptio placentae;
  - fibroid degeneration (usually at mid-trimester).
- Non-obstetric causes:
  - urinary tract infection, pyelonephritis;
  - irritable bowel syndrome, constipation;
  - ovarian cyst (haemorrhage, torsion).

A2 The history seems to suggest preterm labour (uterine contractions) – a diagnosis that will have to be confirmed. There are many causes of preterm labour. Smoking is a risk factor for abruptio placentae which may lead to preterm labour.

A3 The history should first establish whether the uterine activity is regular or irregular. Irregular uterine action is not usually associated with labour (Braxton Hicks contractions). Regular, painful contractions that progressively become longer, more painful and more frequent are typically labour pains. Lack of pain-free intervals would suggest abruptio placentae. Vaginal bleeding is often (but not always, as in concealed abruption) associated with abruptio placentae. A history of ruptured membranes supports the diagnosis of chorionamnionitis. A history of urinary symptoms (dysuria, loin pain, etc.) and bowel symptoms (vomiting, diarrhoea, etc.) might suggest a non-obstetric cause of the problem. Ureteric colic can mimic labour pains. A history of fibroids on scan might suggest red degeneration, especially if the pain is localized.

A4 A general examination, including pulse, temperature and blood pressure, is required. The abdomen should be examined to determine uterine irritability and contractility, and the duration of contractions should be determined and loins examined for tenderness. Symphysio–fundal height should be measured and liquor volume should be clinically assessed. Fetal presentation and lie should be examined (this influences the mode of delivery). Uterine tenderness may be associated with abruptio placentae or chorionamnionitis. Listen to the fetal heart, as abruption (heart rate decelerations) or chorionamnionitis (tachycardia) may affect it. Vaginal examination should be performed under sterile conditions to establish the diagnosis of labour. Labour is more likely if the cervical os is open, if the cervix is effaced (short in length) and if the membranes have ruptured.

A5
- **FBC**   ✓   For anaemia and/or neutrophilia.

- **Urinalysis and culture**   ✓   To exclude urinary tract infection.

- **CTG**   ✓   Cardiotocography to assess fetal well-being. Recording of contractions on antenatal CTG only provides information about their frequency, and not about their intensity.

- **USS**   ✓   Ultrasound to check fetal well-being and assess liquor volume (which may be reduced if membranes are ruptured).

- **Coagulation screen**   ±   If abruptio placenta is suspected.

- **Blood group and cross-match**   ±   If abruptio placenta is suspected.

- **Kleihaur test** $\boxed{\pm}$ If abruptio placenta is suspected and patient is Rh-negative.

- **HVS** $\boxed{\checkmark}$ For infection, particularly if there is vaginal discharge or ruptured membranes.

A6
- In preterm labour, management aims to suppress uterine activity and prolong pregnancy (if the maternal and fetal condition allow this), in order to administer steroids which reduce respiratory distress syndrome. This can be achieved by tocolysis using ritodrine or indomethacin.

- If abruptio placentae is suspected, then it should be managed according to the stability of the maternal haemodynamic system and fetal well-being. Administer steroids, but do not attempt to suppress labour, as this might make the haemorrhage worse. Decide on the mode of delivery bearing in mind maternal condition, progress of labour, and fetal presentation and lie.

- If there is suspected infection, give antibiotics, and augment labour if there is clinical evidence of chorionamnionitis.

- *In-utero* transfer will be required if there are no neonatal intensive-care facilities on site.

- If preterm birth occurs, there is a higher risk of recurrence of preterm labour in subsequent pregnancies.

OSCE counselling case 10.1   I have experienced bleeding in pregnancy. How will I be managed?

An 18-year-old woman has had one episode of unprovoked fresh vaginal bleeding at 28 weeks' gestation. An ultrasound scan shows a normally growing fetus with a placenta sited in the lower segment as Grade I placenta praevia. The patient has no abdominal tenderness. Her cardiotocograph is normal, her haemoglobin is 12.0 g/dL and her blood group is rhesus-negative. She has been in the hospital for a few days and the bleeding has not recurred.

Q1 What information is required for counselling this patient about how she will be managed during the rest of her pregnancy?

OSCE counselling case 10.2   How should I record fetal movements?

A 29-year-old woman presents with reduced fetal movements at 35 weeks' gestation. Investigations show a normal cardiotocograph.

Q1 What information is required for counselling this patient about monitoring her fetal movements over the next few weeks?

OSCE counselling case 10.1 — I have experienced bleeding in pregnancy. How will I be managed?

Answers

- This patient has minor placenta praevia (Grades I and II), which is likely to be the cause of her antepartum haemorrhage.

- There is no need for long-term hospitalization, which would only be necessary for major placenta praevia (Grades III and IV).

- There is no cause for concern, as the bleeding has stopped. However, there is a risk of recurrence and preterm delivery.

- Frequent visits will be required throughout the rest of the pregnancy.

- If there is no further bleeding, placental site and fetal growth should be checked by ultrasound scan at 34 weeks' gestation.

- If there is recurrent bleeding after the patient has been discharged home, she should return to hospital immediately. If there is a risk of preterm birth, steroids should be administered for fetal lung maturity. Tocolysis is generally contraindicated in antepartum haemorrhage.

- Advise against intercourse.

- Anti-D injection will be required.

OSCE counselling case 10.2 — How should I record fetal movements?

Answers

- A kick chart is the established method for monitoring fetal movement.

- This chart reassures the patient that all is well, and allows her to identify potential problems in an objective way.

- Specific instructions on how to use the chart include the following.

  1 Begin at 09.00 hours.

  2 Count every separate movement and record it on the chart with a tick.

  3 If the baby has not moved at least 10 times by 18.00 hours, then the patient should attend the labour suite.

  4 In the labour suite the patient will undergo cardiotocography and other investigations if required.

  5 Further management will depend on the findings of these tests, and they might warrant expediting delivery.

- Smoking, dehydration and poor food intake can reduce fetal movements.

- Warn the patient that, with increasing gestation, the time taken to detect the full 10 movements will become longer. This is normal as long as the 10 movements occur before 18.00 hours.

The clinical cases included in this chapter are as follows:

Case 11.1   My baby is due and I think I am in labour
Case 11.2   I am in labour and the midwife says my baby is getting tired
Case 11.3   The midwife says my labour is not progressing
Case 11.4   The midwife says my labour is not progressing

The OSCE counselling cases included in this chapter are as follows:

OSCE counselling case 11.1   What pain relief should I have in labour?
OSCE counselling case 11.2   I have passed my due date and I am not in labour yet

In order to work through the core clinical cases in this chapter, you will need to understand the following key concepts.

KEY CONCEPTS

Stages of labour

First stage – from the onset of regular painful contractions until full dilatation of the cervix.
Second stage – from full dilatation of the cervix until delivery of the baby.
Third stage – from delivery of the baby until delivery of the placenta.

Fetal lie

The relationship of the long axis of the fetus with that of the mother (e.g. longitudinal/transverse).

Presentation

The part of the fetus which occupies the lower segment of the uterus (e.g. cephalic when the head occupies the lower segment).

Presenting part

The lowest part of the fetus that is palpable on vaginal examination.

Position

The position of the fetal presenting part in the maternal pelvis in relation to the 'denominator'; the occiput in a vertex presentation and the sacrum in a breech presentation (e.g. occipito anterior, sacro posterior).

Vertex

The area of the fetal skull that is bordered by the anterior fontanelle, the posterior fontanelle and the parietal eminences.

Engagement

The state when the widest diameter of the fetal presenting part enters the maternal pelvis.

Station

Descent of the presenting part measured in centimetres above or below the level of the ischial spines.

Attitude

The degree of flexion of the fetal head (e.g. vertex, brow or face).

Moulding

The reduction in the diameters of the fetal head caused by the coming together or overlapping of the sutures in the fetal skull as the head is compressed by the maternal pelvis.

Caput

Localized swelling of the fetal scalp secondary to pressure during labour.

Postpartum haemorrhage

Primary – the loss of > 500 mL of blood within 24 h of delivery.
Secondary – the loss of > 500 mL of blood after 24 h and within 6 weeks of delivery.

Cervical effacement

The length of cervix that shortens to indicate that labour has started. In primiparous women the cervix is tubular and gets 'drawn up' into the lower segment until it is flat.

Bishop score

A measure of the 'favourability' of the cervix for induction of labour. The lower the score, the more unfavourable the cervix.

Points	0	1	2	3	Score
Dilation	0 cm	1–2 cm	3–4 cm	5–6 cm	
Cervical canal length	2 cm	1–2 cm	0.5–1 cm	< 0.5 cm	
Station	−3	−2	−1/0	+1/+2	
Consistency	Firm	Medium	Soft		
Position	Posterior	Mid	Anterior		
				Total	

Case 11.1 My baby is due and I think I am in labour

A 22-year-old primigravida with a singleton pregnancy at term has had an uncomplicated pregnancy. She starts to have regular uterine contractions and telephones the labour suite. On the advice of a midwife, she makes her way to the hospital.

Case 11.2 I am in labour and the midwife says my baby is getting tired

A 20-year-old unemployed single mother has had labour induced at 38 weeks' gestation because the baby was considered to be growth-restricted. This is her first pregnancy, and she smokes 20 cigarettes per day. The cervix is dilated 4 cm, and the midwife is concerned about the cardiotocograph (CTG) (see Figure 11.1)

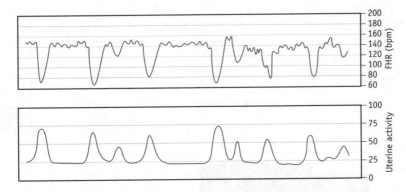

Figure 11.1 *CTG for Case 11.2.*

Case 11.3 The midwife says my labour is not progressing

A 26-year-old primigravida at term is in spontaneous labour. Her height is 172 cm. Her pregnancy has been uncomplicated. She has a singleton pregnancy with a cephalic presentation and the vertex is engaged. She has not required analgesia. Her partogram is shown in Figure 11.2.

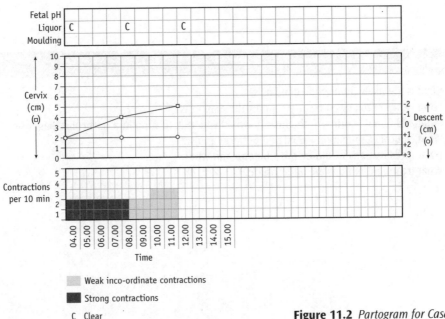

Figure 11.2 *Partogram for Case 11.3.* **123**

Case 11.4   The midwife says my labour is not progressing

A 26-year-old primigravida at term is in spontaneous labour. She has a singleton pregnancy with a longitudinal lie and a cephalic presentation. Her previous pregnancy ended at 34 weeks with a spontaneous vaginal delivery of a 2.0 kg baby. Her height is 150 cm. Her pregnancy has been uncomplicated, but the midwife has often said that 'the baby feels big'. She has been in labour all day and her partogram is shown in Figure 11.3. She has been given oxytocin (syntocinon) for the last 4 h.

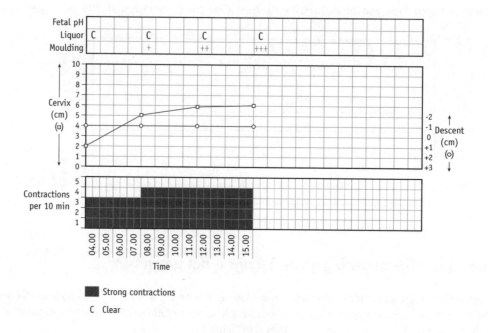

Figure 11.3 *Partogram for Case 11.4.*

Questions *for each of the case scenarios given*

Q1 What is the likely differential diagnosis?
Q2 What issues in the given history support the diagnosis?
Q3 What additional features in the history would you seek to support a particular diagnosis?
Q4 What clinical examination would you perform and why?
Q5 What investigations would be most helpful and why?
Q6 What treatment options are appropriate?

Case 11.1 My baby is due and I think I am in labour

A1
- Labour.
- Braxton Hicks contractions.
- False labour.

A2 Regular uterine contractions at term usually indicate the start of spontaneous labour.

A3 Increasing regularity and duration of contractions would support a diagnosis of the onset of spontaneous labour. A 'show' (mucus plug from the cervix) and/or rupture of the membranes may accompany the onset of labour. A brief history of the current pregnancy should be taken.

A4 A general assessment of maternal condition is made, including measurement of pulse, blood pressure and temperature. Abdominal palpation is performed to feel for uterine contractions, confirm the lie and presentation, check for engagement of the presenting part and listen to the fetal heart. A vaginal examination is performed to check for cervical effacement and dilatation, station and position of the presenting part, and the colour of any liquor draining. Labour would be confirmed if regular uterine contractions were present in association with an effacing and dilating cervix.

A5
- **Urinalysis** ✓ Proteinurea is evidence of pre-eclampsia if associated with raised blood pressure. Ketonuria is evidence of dehydration.

A6
- Maternal well-being should be assessed by regular measurement of the patient's temperature, pulse and blood pressure, which should all be recorded on a partogram. Dehydration should be avoided, with the patient being encouraged to drink water. Because of the delayed gastric emptying time and the risk of aspiration, food should be avoided during labour. The mother should be encouraged to micturate frequently in labour to enable measurement of urine output and to avoid urinary retention. On each occasion the urine can also be tested for protein and ketones.

- Fetal well-being should be assessed by observing the colour of the liquor. The presence of meconium might indicate fetal hypoxia. The fetal heart should be auscultated every 15 min during and for 1 min after a contraction. If an abnormality is detected, or if another indication arises (e.g. epidural analgesia is used), continuous fetal heart rate monitoring should be commenced.

- Progress of labour should be assessed by performing regular (4-hourly) vaginal examinations. The dilatation of the cervix is estimated in centimetres, the descent of the head is measured by its relation to the ischial spines as centimetres above or below an imaginary line drawn between the spines, and these measurements are recorded on a partogram (see Figures 11.2 and 11.3).

- Adequate pain relief should be provided. Transcutaneous electrical nerve stimulation (TENS), entonox, opiates (e.g. pethidine, diamorphine) or an epidural block are commonly used options. The choice will depend on maternal preference in association with factors such as the stage of labour, the availability of an anaesthetist if an epidural is chosen, and other obstetric factors (e.g. hypertension, in which case an epidural may be more appropriate).

Case 11.2 I am in labour and the midwife says my baby is getting tired

A1 Fetal distress in labour.

A2 Fetal growth restriction is a risk factor for fetal hypoxia. The cardiotocography in this case is abnormal, with reduced beat-to-beat variation, no accelerations and variable decelerations.

A3 Additional risk factors for intrauterine growth restriction in which hypoxia is more common include elevated blood pressure, antepartum haemorrhage and chronic maternal disease (e.g. renal disease). Reduced fetal movements may have been noted prior to the induction of labour. Meconium-stained liquor during labour may be associated with fetal hypoxia (see Box 11.1).

A4 Examination would include abdominal palpation, where the fundus may be small for dates. This finding would support fetal growth restriction.

A5 ● **Fetal blood sampling** ☑ The reduced beat-to-beat variation and variable decelerations would give cause for concern (see Box 11.2).

A6 Management would be according to the analysis of fetal blood sampling (see Box 11.3).

Box 11.1 *Intrapartum signs that would indicate fetal distress*

● Meconium staining is present in 15% of all deliveries at term and in 40% of deliveries at post-term.

● Gross meconium staining is likely to be significant and, together with CTG abnormalities, should never be ignored.

● Meconium aspiration by the baby may cause pneumonitis, which can be fatal. Cleaning the upper airway at the time of delivery can prevent this.

Box 11.2 *What should be done when irregularities of the CTG occur?*

Half of all babies who are thought to have 'fetal distress' who are subsequently delivered by forceps or Caesarean section are not hypoxic, and conversely half of the most hypoxic babies do not exhibit classical signs of fetal distress. However, a normal CTG is very reassuring and indicates good fetal well-being.

Under these circumstances CTG monitoring that shows signs of fetal distress should be confirmed by fetal scalp blood sampling to measure fetal pH.

Box 11.3 *Obstetric management following fetal blood sample*

pH < 7.20

Deliver the baby by forceps/ventouse if the cervix is fully dilated and the fetal head is engaged, or by Caesarean section if this is not the case.

pH > 7.20 but < 7.25

Repeat fetal blood sampling after 30 min unless there is a deterioration in CTG prior to this time.

pH > 7.25

Normal result – repeat fetal blood sampling if cardiotocography deteriorates.

Case 11.3   The midwife says my labour is not progressing   Answers

A1 Failure to progress in labour may be due to:
- inadequate uterine activity;
- cephalopelvic disproportion.

A2 Her height (no evidence of short stature) and the fact that the vertex is engaged do not support cephalopelvic disproportion. The lack of requirement for analgesia would support inadequate uterine contractions.

A3 The frequency and duration of contractions should be recorded. Risk factors for cephalopelvic disproportion (e.g. macrosomia, diabetes) should be sought.

A4 Examination would include an abdominal palpation to assess the clinical size of the baby, to assess the amount of head that is palpable in order to determine whether the head is engaged, and also to assess the frequency and strength of uterine contractions. Four-hourly vaginal examinations should be performed to assess the progress of labour, and the findings should be plotted on a partogram (as shown in Figure 11.2). Assessment of fetal position should be made as a malposition (e.g. persistent occipito posterior would create a relative cephalopelvic disproportion because of the increased diameters presented). An assessment of the presence and degree of moulding (overlapping skull bones) and caput (scalp oedema) is required, and would support cephalopelvic disproportion. An assessment of liquor colour should be made, with the presence of meconium indicating the possibility of fetal hypoxia. Maternal well-being (pulse, blood pressure, temperature, urine output) should be assessed and adequate analgesia provided.

A5
- **CTG** ☑ To look for evidence of fetal distress.
- **FBC** ☑ To check for anaemia in case Caesarean section is required.
- **Group and save blood** ☑ In case Caesarean section is required and a transfusion becomes necessary as a result.

A6 Commence oxytocin (syntocinon) and reassess in 4 h if there is still no concern about fetal condition. Oxytocin makes the contractions more regular, stronger and more frequent, resulting in effective uterine contractions that will lead to cervical dilatation and fetal head descent.

Case 11.4 The midwife says my labour is not progressing

A1 Failure to progress in labour may be due to:
- cephalopelvic disproportion;
- poor uterine contractility.

A2 Her height (short stature) and the fact that her baby is clinically large (macrosomic) point towards cephalopelvic disproportion. Her uterine contractions are adequate as recorded on the partogram.

A3 Consider predisposing factors for macrosomia (e.g. gestational diabetes).

A4 Examination would include an abdominal palpation to assess the clinical size of the baby and to assess the amount of fetal head that is palpable in order to determine whether the head is engaged. The frequency and strength of uterine contractions also need to be assessed. Four-hourly vaginal examinations would be performed to assess the progress of labour, and the findings should be plotted on a partogram. At vaginal examination, assessment of the position of the vertex would be required as a malposition (e.g. persistent occipito posterior could create a relative cephalopelvic disproportion because of the increased fetal diameters presented to the maternal pelvis). An assessment should be made of the degree of moulding (overlapping skull bones) and caput (scalp oedema), the presence of which would support cephalopelvic disproportion. The colour of the liquor should be noted, with the presence of meconium indicating the possibility of fetal hypoxia. Assessment should also be made of maternal well-being, and adequate pain relief should be provided.

A5
- **CTG** ☑ To look for evidence of fetal distress.
- **FBC** ☑ To check for anaemia in case Caesarean section is required.
- **Group and save blood** ☑ In case Caesarean section is required and a transfusion becomes necessary as a result.

A6 Caesarean section under spinal or epidural anaesthesia is required because, according to the partogram, the cervix has not dilated for 4 h, the fetal head has not descended in the maternal pelvis, and labour has not progressed despite 4 h of uterine stimulation with oxytocin.

OSCE counselling case 11.1   What pain relief should I have in labour?

A primigravida who is attending her first antenatal clinic wishes to know more about the pain relief that will be available to her during labour.

Q1   What are the options for pain relief during labour?

OSCE counselling case 11.2   I have passed my due date and I am not in labour yet

A primigravida attends her antenatal clinic at 42 weeks. The pregnancy was dated by ultrasound scan in the second trimester, and she has had a normal antenatal course. The fetus is well grown and lying longitudinally with cephalic presentation. The mother wishes to have labour induced. Apart from some irregular uterine contractions, she has not gone into labour spontaneously.

Q1   What information will be required for counselling her about induction of labour for post-term pregnancy?

OSCE counselling case 11.1   What pain relief should I have in labour?

A1

- Antenatal preparation and a calm labour environment are important. The presence of a partner or birth attendant who can rub and/or massage the woman's back and provide reassurance and support can help during labour. Attendance at parentcraft classes will help the woman to prepare for labour.

- Choices of analgesia in labour include the following.

  1 Transcutaneous electrical nerve stimulation (TENS) can be of benefit in early labour.

  2 Entonox inhalation has a rapid onset with mild analgesic effects. Again it is most effective in early labour. It is best to start inhaling before the onset of a contraction and to continue until the end of the contraction. It can cause light-headedness and nausea.

  3 Opiates such as pethidine can be given as an intramuscular injection every 4–6 h. Pethidine has central sedative effects rather than providing effective analgesia. Patients can therefore become confused and feel 'out of control'. It also causes nausea, so there is often a need for anti-emetics. It can cause a sleep pattern in the fetus so the fetal heart rate may show some abnormality. At birth, respiratory depression can also occur in the neonate. Diamorphine given in a similar fashion has a stronger analgesic effect.

  4 Epidural analgesia with or without opiates is a very effective form of analgesia which can be either given intermittently or infused continuously via a pump. It completely blocks sensation (except pressure) and induces partial motor blockade, making the legs feel heavy and 'dead', so mobility is restricted. It is useful if operative delivery is required.

- These options can be tried in the above sequence, or it may be necessary to skip the sequence and use epidural analgesia directly. Many women do not need to go beyond pethidine in the above sequence.

OSCE counselling case 11.2 I have passed my due date and I am not in labour yet
Answers

A1 • Post-term pregnancy occurs in about 10% of pregnant women.

• One approach to management of this condition is to monitor fetal well-being while awaiting spontaneous labour, but it is reasonable to induce labour as an alternative. If the mother wishes for this, one should go along with her wishes.

• On admission to hospital, fetal well-being will be assessed. If all is well, then maternal condition will be assessed.

• The state of the cervix will be examined in order to determine its length, dilatation, consistency and position (a score can be calculated in combination with the station of the fetal head. See Bishop score on page 122). If the cervix is already quite dilated and effaced (short in length), the fetal membranes can be ruptured artificially, which would result in most women going into labour a short time afterwards.

• If the cervix is not dilated and effaced, prostaglandin may be administered in the form of a vaginal gel. The prostaglandin usually softens and effaces the cervix. Sometimes it can start labour off as well. If labour does not begin with this treatment, then a further dose of prostaglandin may be administered, or the fetal membranes may be ruptured artificially.

• If rupturing the membranes does not initiate labour, then the latter may be induced or augmented with oxytocin (syntocinon) infusion.

• If induction of labour fails completely, a Caesarean delivery may be performed.

• If induction of labour is successful, there is a slightly higher probability of fetal heart rate abnormalities in labour, which may lead to a higher probability of the need for Caesarean delivery.

• Labour after successful induction is managed in the usual manner with regard to pain relief.

Box 11.4 *Post-dates pregnancy*

• Perinatal mortality increases by twofold after 42 weeks.
• The Caesarean section rate increases by twofold after 42 weeks.
• Meconium staining occurs in 40% of pregnancies beyond 42 weeks.
• Caesarean section rates increase in association with induction of labour in post-dates pregnancy together with an unripe cervix.

12 Medical disorders of pregnancy

The clinical cases included in this chapter are as follows:
  Case 12.1 I am pregnant and the midwife says my blood pressure is high
  Case 12.2 I am 28 weeks pregnant and have sugar in my urine
  Case 12.3 I am pregnant and I am also anaemic

The OSCE counselling cases included in this chapter are as follows:
  OSCE counselling case 12.1 I am a diabetic and want to become pregnant
  OSCE counselling case 12.2 My epilepsy is under control and I want to become pregnant

Case 12.1 I am pregnant and the midwife says my blood pressure is high

A 20-year-old primigravida attends the antenatal clinic at 34 weeks' gestation and is noted to have a blood pressure of 150/95 mmHg. Urinalysis is negative. Her blood pressure had previously been recorded in the range 130–150/80–85 mmHg in the mid-trimester. The fetus was clinically an appropriate size for dates. Three days later her blood pressure is 160/100 mmHg and she has developed '++' proteinurea on dipstix testing.

Case 12.2 I am 28 weeks pregnant and have sugar in my urine

A 38-year-old woman with two previous normal deliveries is at 28 weeks' gestation. Her weight is 102 kg. Her pregnancy has been progressing well. She attends the antenatal clinic for a routine visit, and on urinalysis is noted to have '+++' glucose in her urine.

Case 12.3 I am pregnant and I am also anaemic

A 28-year-old vegetarian woman attended the antenatal booking clinic at 12 weeks' gestation. Her five children are aged between 6 months and 8 years. Her haemoglobin level was noted to be 8.5 g/dL.

Questions *for each of the case scenarios given*

Q1 What is the likely differential diagnosis?
Q2 What issues in the given history support the diagnosis?
Q3 What additional features in the history would you seek to support a particular diagnosis?
Q4 What clinical examination would you perform and why?
Q5 What investigations would be most helpful and why?
Q6 What treatment options are appropriate?

Case 12.1   I am pregnant and the midwife says my blood pressure is high

A1
- Pre-eclampsia (pregnancy-induced proteinuric hypertension).
- Essential hypertension.
- Hypertension secondary to another medical condition (e.g. renal disease or diabetes).

A2 Pre-eclampsia – based on the fact that the woman's blood pressure is above 140/90 mmHg with significant proteinurea. She is a primigravida, among whom pre-eclampsia is more common.

A3 Any related symptoms (e.g. headache, visual disturbances, epigastric pain) which indicate worsening disease. Past history of medical disorders which might cause hypertension (e.g. renal disease or diabetes). Booking blood pressure to rule out pre-existing essential hypertension.

A4 Examination would include fundoscopy to identify hypertensive retinopathy. The reflexes should be examined to identify hyperreflexia, which would indicate severe pre-eclampsia or impending eclampsia.

A5

• **U&E**	✓	To identify renal compromise.
• **FBC**	✓	A fall in platelet count indicates worsening disease.
• **LFT**	±	If clinically indicated (i.e. worsening blood pressure or increased proteinurea), investigation may include liver function tests to identify the presence of HELLP syndrome (**H**aemolysis, **E**levated **L**iver enzymes and **L**ow **P**latelets).
• **Urinalysis**	✓	Twice daily urinalysis for proteinurea. Twenty-four hour urinary protein may also be measured.
• **USS**	✓	To assess growth and well-being.
• **CTG**	✓	To assess fetal well-being.

A6 Pre-eclampsia is usually a progressive condition. Treatment lies in delivery. In the meantime the aim is to monitor and control blood pressure and to plan delivery as close to fetal maturity as possible. The woman should be admitted to the antenatal ward. Biochemical and haematological assessment should be performed as described above. Regular (at least 4-hourly) blood pressure assessments should be made in order to identify worsening condition. A fluid balance chart should be commenced to identify oliguria. Twice daily urinalysis for proteinurea should be performed. Assessment of fetal condition, including ultrasound biometry, umbilical Doppler and cardiotocography should be undertaken. Maternal steroids should be administered in case early delivery is indicated. Consider starting antihypertensive therapy if systolic blood pressure is greater than 170 mmHg and diastolic pressure is greater than 110 mmHg. This controls blood pressure but does not alter the progression of pre-eclampsia. If there is hyperreflexia and/or HELLP syndrome, delivery is indicated. In this instance, magnesium sulphate may be used to prevent the development of eclampsia.

Box 12.1 *Risks of pre-eclampsia*

Maternal complications:
- eclampsia;
- cerebrovascular accident;
- HELLP syndrome;
- disseminated intravascular coagulation;
- liver failure;
- renal failure;
- pulmonary oedema;
- maternal death.

Fetal complications:
- intrauterine growth restriction;
- placental abruption;
- Fetal death.

Case 12.2   I am 28 weeks pregnant and have sugar in my urine   Answers

A1
- Reduced renal threshold for glucose during pregnancy.
- Gestational diabetes.

A2 The woman's age and her weight increase her risk of gestational diabetes.

A3 Multiple pregnancy, a family history of insulin-dependent diabetes in a first-degree relative, a previous history of gestational diabetes, a previous unexplained intrauterine death, polyhydramnios and a previous large-for-dates baby are all risk factors for gestational diabetes.

A4 Examination should include fundoscopy for diabetic retinopathy and abdominal palpation for evidence of a 'large-for-dates' fetus or polyhydramnios.

A5
- **Glucose**   ☑   A fasting blood glucose concentration of > 5.5 mmol/L and/or a 2-h blood glucose concentration of > 9.0 mmol/L using a 75-g carbohydrate test would confirm the diagnosis of gestational diabetes.

- **Glycosylated haemoglobin**   ☑   To identify long-term hyperglycaemia.

A6 There continues to be much debate about the definition, significance and management of gestational diabetes. However, current recommendations are that women with impaired glucose tolerance should be managed for the remainder of their pregnancy as if they had gestational diabetes.

MANAGEMENT OF GESTATIONAL DIABETES

- Review of the woman's diet to include high levels of complex carbohydrate, soluble fibre and reduced saturated fats. An energy prescription of 30–35 kcal/kg pre-pregnant optimum body weight is ideal, with at least 50% of energy being derived from carbohydrate.

- Preprandial blood glucose monitoring (i.e. 4 times daily) should be commenced. If blood glucose levels are consistently above 6.0–7.0 mmol/L despite adherence to diet, insulin should be commenced. A regime of preprandial short-acting human insulin (three times daily humulin S) and overnight longer-acting insulin (humulin I) should be used. Insulin requirements will increase during pregnancy, and should be adjusted accordingly.

- Measurement of glycosylated haemoglobin every 4–6 weeks is common practice, but has not been shown to improve outcome.

- A retinal examination should be performed every 4–6 weeks.

ANTENATAL CARE

- Ultrasound examination should be performed fortnightly in the third trimester to measure abdominal circumference as an assessment of fetal growth, to assess liquor volume and to perform umbilical arterial Doppler.

- More frequent visits will be necessary to allow optimal management of diabetic control and to screen for complications of pregnancy, which are more common (e.g. proteinuric hypertension).

- A multiprofessional team in a dedicated well-organized diabetic antenatal clinic should assume responsibility for care. The team should include an obstetrician with an interest in diabetes in pregnancy, a diabetic physician, a midwife, diabetic nurse and a dietitian.

TIMING AND MODE OF DELIVERY

- With good diabetic control and in the absence of obstetric complications, delivery at term and by the vaginal route should be the aim.

- Women with gestational diabetes who are on insulin require an insulin and dextrose infusion, aiming to keep blood sugar levels between 4.0 and 6.0 mmol/L. Blood glucose levels should be checked hourly. Women who are controlled by diet do not need to monitor blood glucose levels during labour.

- Effective pain relief is important, and an epidural should be considered.

- Continual fetal heart rate monitoring should be used because of the increased risk of fetal distress.

- It is important to be aware of the increased risk of shoulder dystocia and to take appropriate precautions at delivery (i.e. maternal position (consider lithotomy) and episiotomy, particularly if the scans suggest that the fetus is large-for-dates).

POSTNATAL CARE

- For women who are on insulin, this should be stopped following delivery of the placenta.

- Breastfeeding should be encouraged.

- Prophylactic antibiotics should be given at the time of Caesarean section if required.

- All gestational diabetics should be seen at 6 weeks for a postnatal check and glucose tolerance test. In most women this will be normal, but they remain at risk of developing diabetes in the future (40–50% of cases). They should all therefore be given general advice about weight and diet, and should have annual fasting blood glucose tests for early detection of diabetes.

Box 12.2 *Risks of gestational diabetes*

Risks of gestational diabetes for the mother include:
- macrosomia and a difficult delivery (shoulder dystocia or the need for Caesarean section for cephalopelvic disproportion);
- polyhydramnios;
- risk of the mother developing diabetes in the future.

Risks of gestational diabetes for the baby include:
- hypoglycaemia;
- hypocalcaemia;
- palsies and fractures due to difficult delivery.

A1
- Iron-deficiency anaemia.
- Sickle-cell disease.
- Thalassaemia.
- Folate deficiency.

A2 Iron-deficiency amaemia is supported by the woman's high parity and narrow spacing between children. This is the commonest type of anaemia in pregnancy, affecting approximately 10% of women. Her vegetarian diet would predispose to reduced iron intake.

A3 An additional history would include symptoms (e.g. tiredness, breathlessness, 'light-headedness or dizziness'), a previous history of anaemia, the use of iron supplements and the patient's country of origin. Symptoms of anaemia are usually absent unless the haemoglobin concentration is less than 8 g/dL. Around 10% of Afro-Caribbeans in the UK are heterozygous for sickle-cell disease, and thalassaemia is most prevalent in individuals from the Mediterranean region and South-East Asia.

A4 Examination would include a search for evidence of pallor (generally the sclera and palms) and abdominal examination for hepatosplenomegaly.

A5

• **Blood film**	✓	Microcytosis and hypochromia can be seen on blood film. Hypersegmented neutrophils are seen in folate deficiency.
• **FBC**	✓	Both mean cell volume (MCV) and mean cell haemoglobin (MCH) are reduced in iron-deficiency anaemia. MCV is usually increased in folate deficiency. Haemoglobin estimation in pregnancy should not be the only parameter to be assessed as a sign of anaemia, as it can be lowered as a result of haemodilution. If the MCV is in the normal range then this would signify haemodilution, and if microcytosis is present an iron deficiency or haemoglobinopathy is likely.
• **Ferritin levels**	✓	Ferritin levels should be measured if microcytosis is present. Levels are reduced in iron-deficiency anaemia.
• **Red-cell folate**	±	Red-cell folate should be measured if anaemia is present without marked microcytosis.
• **Sickledex test and haemoglobin electrophoresis**	±	Sickledex test and if positive haemoglobin electrophoresis for sickle-cell trait. If the woman is sickledex positive, her partner should be tested and appropriate counselling given about the prenatal diagnosis.
• **Haemoglobin A2**	±	Haemoglobin A2 quantitation is required for thalassaemia, and again if a positive result is obtained the partner should be tested.

A6 Iron-deficiency anaemia should be treated with iron supplementation. The rarer folate deficiency should be treated with folate supplementation. The aim should be to correct anaemia before delivery. However, as folic acid reduces the risk of neural-tube defects, it should be recommended to all women.

- Heterozygous sickle-cell carriers usually have no problems and do not require treatment. They may in extreme situations (e.g. hypoxia, infections) develop 'crises'. Homozygotes are likely to have been affected by 'crises' and have chronic haemolytic anaemia all their lives. In pregnancy they have increased perinatal mortality and are at risk of thrombosis, infection and sickle 'crises'. Treatment includes exchange transfusions, screening for infection, folic acid and avoidance of precipitating factors for crises. Iron should be avoided.

- For women with heterozygous alpha-thalassaemia, iron and folate supplementation are required. In beta-thalassaemia, heterozygous women have a chronic anaemia which can worsen during pregnancy. They may require transfusion. Pregnancy in homozygous individuals is uncommon. However, in these cases folic acid is required but iron should be avoided.

OSCE counselling case 12.1   I am a diabetic and want to become pregnant

A 23-year-old insulin-dependent diabetic is taking the combined oral contraceptive pill. She wants to come off the pill to try for a pregnancy.

Q1   What pre-pregnancy counselling would you provide for this woman?

OSCE counselling case 12.2   My epilepsy is under control and I want to become pregnant

A 26-year-old woman who is an epileptic controlled on treatment is planning to get married. She is concerned about pregnancy and her epileptic medication. She has been seizure-free for 6 years on two anti-epileptic drugs. She has not recently been reviewed by a neurologist.

Q1   What pre-pregnancy care and counselling would you give this woman?

OSCE counselling case 12.1   I am a diabetic and want to become pregnant

- The diabetic control should be optimized before pregnancy in order to reduce the risk of congenital anomalies. If the patient is not regularly monitoring her blood sugar levels, this would need to be commenced with the aim of adjusting insulin to keep preprandial levels to between 4 and 7 mmol/L. A glycosylated haemoglobin concentration would give an indication of longer-term control.

- The provision of glucagon would need to be checked because of the increased risk of hypoglycaemic attacks with the tighter control. It would be important for the woman's partner to know when and how to administer the glucagon.

- Commence folic acid supplementation to reduce the risk of neural-tube defects.

- Check whether the woman is rubella immune, and give immunization prior to stopping the pill if she is not.

- Emphasize the need to report early after a missed period to ensure early referral to a specialist antenatal clinic.

- Arrange an eye examination to identify pre-existing retinopathy, which should be treated prior to pregnancy.

OSCE counselling case 12.2 My epilepsy is under control and I want to become pregnant

A1

- The majority of babies who are born to epileptic mothers are normal. However, women with epilepsy, particularly those taking anti-epileptic drugs, are at increased risk of giving birth to a baby with congenital anomalies (e.g. neural-tube defects).

- Before and during pregnancy, the aim should be to prescribe the lowest dose and number of anti-epileptic drugs necessary to protect against seizures. Suggest referral to a neurologist to consider pre-pregnancy withdrawal of anti-epileptic drugs or a change to monotherapy.

- Emphasize the importance of periconceptual folic acid.

- Recommend serum αFP screening and a detailed ultrasound scan at 18–20 weeks to identify fetal anomalies.

- Check whether the woman is rubella immune, and provide immunization if appropriate.

13 Puerperium

The clinical cases included in this chapter are as follows:
Case 13.1   My baby has just delivered amd I am bleeding heavily
Case 13.2   I had a baby 3 days ago and I feel shivery
Case 13.3   The midwife is concerned because I have little interest in my baby

The OSCE counselling cases included in this chapter are as follows:
OSCE counselling case 13.1   Should I be breastfeeding my baby?
OSCE counselling case 13.2   My baby has breathing difficulties after Caesarean birth

Case 13.1   My baby has just delivered and I am bleeding heavily

A 36-year-old woman with five children and a history of previous short labours delivered her baby 10 min ago. She had been in labour on this occasion for 12 h after a spontaneous onset. She continues to bleed heavily.

Case 13.2   I had a baby 3 days ago and feel shivery

A 34-year-old primiparous woman had a traumatic vaginal delivery after an 18-h labour. Labour was induced after pre-labour rupture of the membranes for over 48 h. Three days post-delivery the woman feels shivery and has had a temperature of 38.4°C and 38.5°C measured 4 h apart. She is a smoker, but had stopped smoking during pregnancy.

Case 13.3   The midwife is concerned because I have little interest in my baby

An elderly primigravida feels that she has very little interest in her baby 3 days post delivery. She is a solicitor by profession, and became pregnant after assisted conception. The pregnancy and delivery were uneventful. There is no past history or family history of mental illness.

Questions *for each of the case scenarios given*

Q1   What is the likely differential diagnosis?
Q2   What issues in the given history support the diagnosis?
Q3   What additional features in the history would you seek to support a particular diagnosis?
Q4   What clinical examination would you perform and why?
Q5   What investigations would be most helpful and why?
Q6   What treatment options are appropriate?

Case 13.1 My baby has just delivered and I am bleeding heavily Answers

A1 Primary postpartum haemorrhage:
- atonic uterus, with or without retained placenta or placental segments;
- cervical, vaginal or perineal trauma.

A2 Grand multiparity and prolonged labour are both risk factors for postpartum haemorrhage.

A3 A history of induced labour, retained placenta, previous postpartum haemorrhage, operative delivery, polyhydramnios, multiple pregnancy, antepartum haemorrhage, previous Caesarean section or a coagulation defect would all increase this woman's risk of postpartum haemorrhage.

A4 Examination would include measurement of pulse and blood pressure for evidence of shock. An assessment of blood loss and continuing loss is required. Abdominal examination would include palpation of the uterine fundus to look for a poorly contracted uterus. A check for obvious vaginal/perineal trauma should be made, and the midwife should be asked to check the completeness of the placenta.

A5
- **FBC** ✓ To identify anaemia and platelet count.

- **Blood cross-match** ✓ To replace blood loss and treat shock.

- **Clotting screen** ✓ To identify a coagulopathy.

A6
- Initial management should be to obtain intravenous access and commence IV fluids. The uterine fundus should be 'rubbed up' if it is not contracted. An IV syntocinon infusion should be commenced and IM/IV ergometrine given to contract the uterus. Any vaginal or perineal trauma should be sutured.

- If the bleeding continues, manage shock and call for senior obstetric and anaesthetic assistance. Give oxygen, insert a further large-gauge venflon and commence colloid and/or blood when cross-matched, or O-negative blood. Ensure that an adequate request has been made for cross-matched blood (at least 8 units) and check clotting. Continue to compress the uterus bimanually if it is not contracted. Continue the IV infusion of syntocinon. Consider giving rectal, IM or intramyometrial prostaglandin. Catheterize the patient to monitor urine output, and insert a central venous pressure line. If the bleeding persists, examine under an anaesthetic to check that the uterine cavity is empty of retained products of conception, and to identify and suture any trauma to the cervix, vagina or perineum. If bleeding still persists, consider a laparotomy with ligation of the internal iliac arteries, or hysterectomy.

Case 13.2   I had a baby 3 days ago and feel shivery   Answers

A1
- Endometritis.
- Perineal wound infection.
- Breast infection/abscess.
- Urinary tract infection.
- Chest infection.
- Deep venous thrombosis.

A2 Delivery associated with perineal lacerations has a high probability of developing infection due to perineal cross-infection. A prolonged labour with ruptured membranes and repeated vaginal examinations during induction of labour can result in endometritis. Smoking is also a risk factor for chest infection. Symptoms of shivers and a temperature indicate an infection. However, a maternal pyrexia of > 38°C is not usually associated with deep venous thrombosis, which causes a low-grade pyrexia.

A3 For endometritis, the lochia may be offensive. A history of frequency and dysuria may indicate urinary tract infection, which is a common cause of postpartum pyrexia. If the patient is also catheterized during labour, this can lead to urinary tract infection. An enquiry should be made to ensure that the placenta was complete at the third stage of labour, to exclude infection of a retained placenta. This history may not be diagnostic.

A4 Pulse, blood pressure, peripheral perfusion and signs of cyanosis should be sought. Examination is required of the chest, breasts (enlargment, warmth and tenderness and a fluctuant tender mass together with enlarged axillary lymph nodes may be due to an abscess), abdomen (to check for involution of the uterus), loins (for renal tenderness), intravenous access sites and legs (for swelling and tenderness). Vulval examination of the perineal wound would also be mandatory. A vaginal examination should be performed to determine whether the cervical os is open. It may indicate retained products and an enlarged tender uterus. If the patient had a Caesarean section, then a wound haematoma infection or abscess would need to be excluded.

A5
- **FBC**   ☑   Blood for white cell count – increased polymorphs would indicate infection.
- **HVS and**   ☑   For culture and sensitivity testing for infection.
  endocervical swabs
- **Urine culture** ☑   To exclude a urinary tract infection.
- **Blood cultures** ☑   To exclude septicaemia in view of the patient's high temperature.
- **Chest X-ray**   ☑   To exclude a chest infection.
- **Ultrasound**   ☑   To exclude a deep venous thrombosis.
  Doppler analysis of leg veins

A6
- Manage sepsis aggressively with a microbiologist's input.

- Endometritis – augmentin and metronidazole or erythromycin and metronidazole (covers anaerobes).

- *Urinary tract infection* – cephalosporins, penicillins/augmentin (covers Gram-negative cocci). Increase fluid intake.

- *Perineal wound infection* – administer broad-spectrum antibiotics which should include metronidazole. Keep the wound clean and dry to allow rapid healing. If an abscess is present, any sutures should be cut to allow the abscess to drain.

- *Breast infection/abscess* – stop breastfeeding from the affected breast, but still continue to express the milk. Administer penicillins/broad-spectrum antibiotics.

- Incise and drain if there is an obvious abscess.

- *Chest infection* – chest physiotherapy, and amoxycillin/augmentin (covers Gram-positive cocci).

- *Deep venous thrombosis/pulmonary embolism* – pulmonary embolism is a leading cause of maternal mortality. Half the deaths are postnatal, usually occurring after discharge from hospital. Early mobility and hydration are important preventative measures for all postnatal women.

Management of deep venous thrombosis and pulmonary embolism should be arranged in collaboration with the physicians so that the appropriate anticoagulant regime is administered. Risk markers should be tested at 6 weeks' postpartum (i.e. protein S & C deficiency, factor V Leidin mutation and antithrombin III levels).

Case 13.3 The midwife is concerned because I have little interest in my baby

A1
- Postpartum 'baby blues'.
- Depression.
- Puerperal psychosis.

A2
In most cases with the given history there is no psychiatric problem, as minor psychological symptoms are common after birth. Postpartum 'baby blues' are at their worst around the third to fifth day after the birth, but resolve by about the tenth day. However, this case needs further investigation in order to exclude major psychosis or depression, particularly if the symptoms occur later, around 4–6 weeks after birth. Lack of family history and past history of mental illness supports a benign transient phenomenon, but the woman's advanced age, higher social class, primigravidity and infertility treatment are all risk factors for major mental illness.

A3
The history should explore psychological symptoms such as variation in mood, poor sleep, weeping, lethargy, irritability, hallucinations, delusions, etc. Operative mode of delivery, multiple pregnancy and complications during pregnancy all increase the likelihood of major mental illness.

A4
A mental state examination is required.

A5
- **TFT** ☑ Thyrotoxicosis should be excluded if major mental illness is suspected.

A6
- Postpartum blues – psychological support and reassurance should be offered.

- Refer the patient to a psychiatrist if depression or psychosis is suspected. Early diagnosis is important, as it can interfere with mother–baby bonding.

- Depression – antidepressants (e.g. imipramine, which does not interfere with breastfeeding).

- Puerperal psychosis – admission to a psychiatric ward is essential, as there is a risk of suicide. The mother should be separated from the baby as there is a risk of neglect and harm. Neuroleptics may be used.

OSCE counselling case 13.1   Should I be breastfeeding my baby?

A primigravida has just delivered a healthy 3600 g baby.

Q1   What are the advantages and disadvantages of breastfeeding?

OSCE counselling case 13.2   My baby has breathing difficulties after Caesarean birth

A baby has been admitted to the neonatal unit with breathing difficulties following a Caesarean section at term because of failure to progress. There was no fetal distress or birth asphyxia. The baby started grunting at 30 min of age. Clinical examination and X-ray suggest transient tachypnoea of the newborn (TTN).

Q1   Explain to the mother what is wrong with her baby and how it will be managed.

A1 Advantages include the following:

- no cost;

- no risk of infection from bottles;

- breast milk contains protein, fat and solute content 'designed' for babies (i.e. appropriate nutritional content);

- contraceptive when fully breastfeeding;

- provides protection against infection (by providing passive immunity via maternal antibodies) and allergies in neonate;

- reduced respiratory and gastrointestinal illness in the child;

- infant–mother bonding is promoted;

- protection against maternal breast, endometrial and ovarian cancer;

- rapid reduction in maternal weight gained from pregnancy;

- effect on child development (e.g. potentially improved cognitive function).

Disadvantages include the following:

- breast milk jaundice is more common;

- can lead to maternal exhaustion, as it involves feeding on demand;.

- can cause pain/discomfort due to breast engorgement;

- leaking of milk from breasts may occur;

- without good support/encouragement, particularly in the early days when establishing breastfeeding, there is a greater likelihood of giving up due to poor milk flow.

Despite these minor disadvantages, all mothers should be encouraged to breastfeed their babies.

OSCE counselling case 13.2   My baby has breathing difficulties after Caesarean birth

A1   Transient tachypnoea of the newborn (TTN):

- a benign transient problem with recovery within 1–2 days;

- a problem of retained lung fluid;

- managed with supportive treatment such as oxygen and intravenous fluids;

- antibiotics can be prescribed, but are not always necessary;

- there are no long-term sequelae;

- the differential diagnosis is of either infection or respiratory distress syndrome (RDS).

OSCE MARKING SCHEME

An example of how counselling stations are marked is given below. This indicates that the content of the answer is not dependent on the factual regurgitation of information, but it includes the assessment of the student's capacity to counsel and communicate with the patient using appropriate terminology. This should be done in a systematic manner so that the patient understands the nature of the consultation.

1. **Introduction**	**1 mark**
2. **Explanation**	**5 marks**

Give 0 marks if not attempted, 0.5 marks if information was given following questioning from the mother, and 1.0 mark if information was given spontaneously

Retained lung fluid	0 – 0.5 – 1.0
Supportive treatment (oxygen, intravenous fluids ± antibiotics)	0 – 0.5 – 1.0
Benign/complete recovery within 1–2 days	0 – 0.5 – 1.0
No sequelae	0 – 0.5 – 1.0
Differential diagnosis: infection, RDS	0 – 0.5 – 1.0
3. **Rapport with patient**	**3 marks**
Non-medical language/terminology	0 – 0.5 – 1.0
Opportunity for patient to ask questions	0 – 0.5 – 1.0
Appropriate pace of consultation	0 – 0.5 – 1.0
4. **Mother's assessment**	**3 marks**
Did you understand the problem after the consultation?	0 – 0.5 – 1.0
Did you have confidence in the candidate?	0 – 0.5 – 1.0
Would you like to see him/her again if he/she was your GP?	0 – 0.5 – 1.0
	TOTAL MARK 12

Index

Index

Vertex 121
Viral warts 41
Virilism 11, 14
Vomiting in pregnancy 85, 90–1

Warts, genital 41
Withdrawal method, contraception 71

Yupze regimen 70